The Silent Enemy

The Silent Enemy
Canada and the
Deadly Flu of 1918

Eileen Pettigrew

Western Producer Prairie Books
Saskatoon, Saskatchewan

Printed and bound in Canada by
Modern Press ◁◆▷1
Saskatoon, Saskatchewan

Cover design by John Luckhurst/GDL

Western Producer Prairie Book publications are produced and manufactured in the middle of Western Canada by a unique publishing venture owned by a group of prairie farmers who are members of Saskatchewan Wheat Pool. From the first book published in 1954, a reprint of a serial originally carried in the weekly newspaper, *The Western Producer*, to the book before you now, the tradition of providing enjoyable and informative reading for all Canadians is continued.

The publisher acknowledges the support received for this publication from the Canada Council.

The publisher has endeavoured to obtain permission to reproduce illustrative material which appears in this book. Any errors or omissions which are brought to the publisher's attention will be rectified in future editions.

Canadian Cataloguing in Publication Data

Pettigrew, Eileen, 1929—
    The silent enemy

Includes index.
Bibliography: p.139
ISBN 0-88833-104-5

1. Influenza — Canada. 2. Influenza — Canada — History. I. Title.
RC150.55.C3P47   614.5'18   C83-091272-X

For Stu

Contents

Contents

Foreword

In the fall of 1918 I was in Toronto with three friends from the University of Alberta, beginning our training in the Royal Air Force as pilots. We were all champing at the bit and eagerly headed for heroes' careers as fighter pilots at the front, in the wake of other young men from the prairie. Our thoughts were on such aces as Billy Bishop, "Wop" May, and Punch Dickens, and not at all of being shot down, and certainly not of dying from the 'flu. Although the influenza epidemic was just beginning to take its heavy toll in eastern Canada, especially amongst Canadian citizen-soldiers returning from, or on the way to, the front, none of us gave a serious thought to the possibility that we might succumb to it.

It was cold in Toronto, especially in the R.A.F. recruits' depot which was then housed in the Jesse Ketchum school on Davenport Road. The sleeping bunks were of the best pine but, alas, had no vestige of mattress or palliasse. I was glad to don heavy issue underwear, however scratchy, and to use at night the thick gray blankets to soften the boards.

We recruits were too many at the time and, although basic training began at once, it was soon interrupted by fatigue duties on the spot or at other camps, such as the flying camp at Beamsville.

In the meantime the epidemic became a very personal experience. Almost daily we were sent with other recruits to the base military hospital, a wooden building on Church or Gerrard Street. It was built and furnished to accommodate three hundred patients, but by then was overcrowded with nine hundred or more. We worked as orderlies, taking out used blankets for fumigation, stretcher-bearing the sick, and carrying out the dead. This is no exaggeration; the toll in one day in October was as many as twelve.

It was not long before the other three left their fatigue duties for the patients' beds. Being lonely for them and miserable with the pine board bunks and duties, I began to think of the more comfortable hospital beds and the sympathetic ministrations of the nurses in white. In this frame of mind I turned up hopefully on sick parade. The first two visits the medical officer said "No." The next day, however, I really had the fever and was sent off to the familiar base hospital, and a bed in the corridor.

Of the next two or three days I have almost no recollection. I must have slept continuously until the fever subsided. I was soon sufficiently over the crisis to be sent for convalescence to the East House of the residences of University College. For ten peaceful days I enjoyed a life of ease, until I was well enough to go on happily with my routine training at Long Branch.

I was at Long Branch when the first false news of an armistice was reported. I easily got a pass and spent a day with two of my friends in the Beamsville camp, actually flying with a very considerate and acrobatic flying officer named Killam. I ended the day in Hamilton, which was delirious with peace celebrations. The next weekend brought the real armistice of November 11, and leave to join the fun in Toronto. The outburst of joy and relief was almost beyond expression.

In a few weeks I was home in Red Deer for Christmas, and in January I was back at the university, a survivor at least, and some sort of veteran, of both the war and the 'flu, without time to think much of what had happened to Canada, or what was happening to other veterans of both these momentous events. It was only later, in retrospect, that I appreciated what Canadians and much of the world had suffered from the dreadful combination of war and pestilence.

The following extract is from my mother's memoirs and gives her experience of the epidemic of 1918:

> The war still dragged along. In April, 1918, Roland was eighteen, and a grown man. He wished to enlist in the Air

Force, and we could not say no. Accordingly, he and his three chums . . . left for Toronto to train. They had not been there long, when the terrible "Flu" epidemic began to sweep over America. The poor boys were all down with it in Camp. Those were anxious days, until we knew they were better. They all recovered. Then our attention was turned to our own household. The flu had reached the West. Everywhere families were down. Schools, churches and places of entertainment were closed. In Alberta we were compelled by law to wear *masks* over our mouths when we went in public. No nurses were to be had, the doctors were overworked, and it looked pretty blue. One by one our little flock took sick, though they were inoculated in the schools. It did no good. . . .

Fortunately neither Father nor I took the disease, but we were nursing night and day, and we brought them safely through. One symptom was the terrific bleeding from the nose. We were so thankful we were spared to nurse our children. I never had any fear of the flu, and right here I wish to express the opinion, that *fear* was one thing that made the epidemic worse. If you are not *afraid* of disease you are *not apt to take it.*

"After a day of cloud and wind and rain, sometimes the setting sun breaks forth again."

So it was in the lives of the people of Canada. After four weary years of bloodshed, after months of disease with all its anxiety and suffering, suddenly, like a great wave of joy, the news of the "Armistice" spread from Atlantic to Pacific. No one, now living, can forget that day — the joy, the ecstacy, the deep thankfulness to God. Father and I could not go down to the town square to help celebrate, as our little ones were too weak yet to be left. But we watched from our hill, and saw the crowds and heard the shouts, and bells ringing. The war was over!! Yes, the *World* war was over!

On November 11th, at 11 A.M., 1918, the war ended. . . . Now we began to think of our soldier boy's return from Toronto. Before Christmas he came, and I think that must have been the happiest Christmas ever, though on many a home lay a shadow that no yuletide cheer could lift.

Eileen Pettigrew's researches and anecdotal history of the Spanish Influenza in Canada took my mind back sixty-five years, to the last three months of World War I.

The Right Honorable Roland Michener

Preface

The factual background for this book came from three main sources: archives and libraries, newspapers of the year 1918, and recollections of individuals. From the first two I have tried to draw a balanced picture of the way people in authority dealt with the crisis, and from the third I sought to show the experiences, reactions, and feelings of Canadians.

Parliament was not sitting during the epidemic, and to my disappointment I found almost nothing relevant in the papers of Prime Minister Robert Laird Borden. He had gone to Britain in November 1918 to head the Canadian delegation to the Peace Conference, and when he returned to Canada the following May, the worst was over in southern Canada. There are, however, reports and letters in the holdings of the Public Archives of Canada and of provincial archives. It is impossible to avoid a feeling of sympathy for officials, preoccupied as they were with the events of World War I and caught up in an emergency for which they were ill-equipped and unprepared. They had to cope the best way they could.

For personal recollections, I wrote to newspapers asking for replies from readers who remembered the time and who would share their reminiscences for a proposed book. Their response was overwhelming. They searched the files of their local newspapers and the holdings of community museums, and contacted friends and relatives. They told me their own memories, not only of the epidemic but of their lives in 1918, and added that if I needed more detail they would be glad to tell me what they could.

They dug through boxes and trunks to find snapshots, sometimes scraping them off album pages. Cameras were not as common then as they are today, and during the emergency people were occupied with more pressing concerns than the taking of pictures. But, if there are few photographs, records of neighbor helping neighbor are vivid still in the minds and hearts of the people who were there. In all the stories that were told to me, one central theme stands out — human kindness.

In all, I corresponded with more than two hundred Canadians from Newfoundland to British Columbia. Assistance from the Explorations Programme of the Canada Council, for which I express my appreciation, helped me to visit personally with many of the people who wrote to me. When recounting the memories of married women, I have identified them by both maiden and married names to avoid any confusion. I wish I could have used every experience described to me, each of which helped me to visualize the events of that troubled time. I am grateful to all those people whose recollections made this book possible, to archivists who went out of their way to help, and to Dr. Andrew J. Rhodes, former professor of microbiology at the University of Toronto and co-author of *Virus Diseases of Man*, who kindly read portions of this manuscript in draft form and made helpful suggestions.

Introduction

In the autumn of 1918, Canada had a population of only about eight million. Out of this small number, it would count nearly sixty thousand dead in World War I, the conflict that H.G. Wells had called "the war that will end war." On the home front, every ounce of energy was directed toward the war effort and there was little time to think about the influenza epidemic that was already sweeping much of the world. When it came, inevitably, to this country, it seemed like the usual winter siege of colds. It was not. It was a killer, and in only a few dread-filled months that fall and winter, between thirty thousand and fifty thousand Canadians were destined to be its victims.

Four Years and More of War

The Canada of 1918 was a different world. Most households did not have telephones, commercial radio was still in the future, and of course there was no television. Saskatchewan men could buy a tailored suit for twenty-three dollars. In Toronto, Ontario, unwrapped bread was delivered to the door by horse and wagon for five cents a loaf, and a teacher in a one-roomed Prince Edward Island school was paid eighteen dollars a month. *Maclean's,* "Canada's National Magazine," featuring writings by Stephen Leacock and Robert W. Service, sold for twenty cents a copy or two dollars a year.

The country had been at war for more than four years, and feelings of patriotism and loyalty to the Mother Country were strong. With the announcement on August 4, 1914 from the British Foreign Office, closing with the words: "His Majesty's Government has declared to the German Government that a state of war exists between Great Britain and Germany from 11 o'clock P.M. August 4," Canadians fell over each other in their eagerness to enlist. Some walked miles to a recruitment centre, and as they boarded trains for camp, it was to the accompaniment of cheers and the playing of bands. Women, who would not have the vote until 1917 and even then only if they were nursing sisters or had close relatives in the service, had to give written permission before their husbands could enlist. Few demurred.

At the outset, Canada's permanent military strength consisted of a regular force of only three thousand and a regular naval complement of three hundred. She had no air force of her own, but Canadian squadrons were formed and one-quarter of Great Britain's air force, about twenty-two thousand officers and men, were Canadian. Near the end of the war, a Royal Canadian Naval Service was formed, and the naval force grew to a total of five thousand.

Despite the small ready-to-go contingent, Canada immediately offered an expeditionary force, and in less than a month more than thirty thousand officers and men were at Valcartier, Quebec, ready to sail for England. Their hearts high with confidence that they could beat the hated Hun and be home for Christmas, their only fear was that it would all be over before they got there. "Britain Called Kaiser's Bluff, Forcing Issue," said the Halifax *Morning Chronicle*; the *Globe* in Toronto headlined: "King George says the Navy Will Revive Its Glories in Action"; Montreal's *Le Devoir* said: "La Guerre"; and in Victoria, the *Daily Colonist* said simply: "Canadians are ready to serve."

Doctors went to war, and so did nurses. Boys left school early to take over the work of the men who were at the Front, and women assumed jobs traditionally held by men. Everyone lent a hand. Rationing was cheerfully accepted by the vast majority, and victory gardens sprang up everywhere.

The Canada Food Board ordered householders to keep on hand only enough flour to be reasonably required for sixty days, unless they lived in very isolated places when they could keep enough for two hundred days. Three residents of the Chaplain district of Saskatchewan were not considered to qualify for the "isolation" requirement and were issued with summonses for hoarding 3,400 pounds of flour and 280 pounds of sugar. The *Swan River Star & Times* in Manitoba exhorted: "Eat less bread!" The butter allowance was two pounds each per month.

Tight hobble skirts worn with high-laced or buttoned boots were the mode for women. A prominent boot-making firm urged its customers to be aware of the need to provide the forces overseas with millions of pairs of shoes. "To this necessity, fashion must yield. We must be content with fewer superfluous styles which serve no useful purpose, but are created merely to look 'different,' " they reminded the readers of their advertisements.

Newsprint was in short supply. Publishers of daily newspapers, of which there were more than there are today, met in Ottawa with R.A. Pringle, controller of newsprint, and agreed to cancel special editions and contests. Government reports were cut drastically; Royal North West Mounted Police reports, for example, dropped from two hundred pages to twenty-five.

While they waited for their men to come home from the Great War, Canadians kept their spirits up by singing "Over There,"

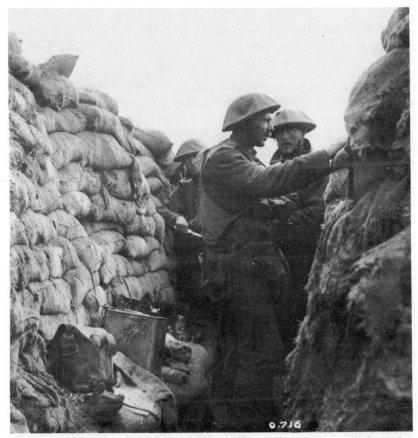

Soldiers in the trenches in the Great War. These fighting men, coming together under adverse conditions, were ready victims of the epidemic. When they returned home, they carried with them the germ of the disease which spread quickly among civilian populations. (Photo courtesy Public Archives Canada, PA 556)

"Soldiers of the Queen," "Peg o' my Heart," and "It's a Long Way to Tipperary." On the battlefields of Germany, France, and Belgium, troops from every corner of the earth stood waist-deep in wet trenches and slogged through mud and snow; they were tired, underfed, cold, and bedevilled by frostbite, trenchfoot, and lice.

Then, as though the world had not enough to contend with, there came a foe that attacked both sides equally, a virulent form of disease that cut down the troops and sent them behind the lines to first-aid stations and hospitals. During May 1918 the British fleet, with 10,313 sailors sick, was too disabled to leave port. King George V was stricken, as were Crown Prince Max of Baden, imperial chancellor of Germany, and the American assistant secretary of the navy, Franklin Delano Roosevelt. Prince Erik of Sweden died of the malady.

The adage "after war comes plague" seemed very apt. These fighting men, coming together under such adverse conditions, were ready victims. For Gordon Stepler of Strathroy, Ontario, serving in France with the Fourth Battery Canadian Field Artillery, the illness was not serious or lengthy. In late June his unit had moved behind the lines for a rest and special training for the expected offensive, and on the twenty-second of the month everyone in the unit came down with 'flu. "It was a quiet time," he remembers. "Both sides were sick." The illness may even have shortened the war. In October 1918, one hundred and eighty thousand cases of influenza were reported in the German army.

The insidious affliction attracted all manner of names, most of them attributing blame to some other nationality. The British troops called it Flanders Grippe; to the Spanish it was Naples Soldier; the Ceylonese called it Bombay Fever; and in Penang it was Singapore Fever. In Hong Kong it was "too much inside sickness," the Germans dubbed it *Blitz Katarrh*, or lightning cold, to the Japanese it was Wrestler's Fever, and in Persia it was called the Disease of the Wind. The Swiss named it The Coquette because it passed its favors around so freely; in Siam it was the Great Cold Fever; in Poland, the Bolshevik Disease; and in Hungary, the Black Whip. To the Royal College of Physicians in Britain it was Spanish Influenza, a name eventually adopted by most of the world.

"Influenza," from the Italian word for influence, had been used to describe disease since the Middle Ages, when it was believed that disease came from the influence of the stars. But "Spanish"? Although eight million Spaniards fell victim, one of them King Alfonso XIII, almost certainly the disease did not begin in that country. It probably started in February 1918 in China, appearing later in France, in the United States during March, in Britain in April, and not in Spain until May; but Spain, being neutral, had no censorship of its press as did countries at war and made the first public announcement of the epidemic in a cable from Madrid to London: "A strange form of disease of epidemic character has appeared in Madrid." Also, Spain's neutrality made her unpopular with both sides, so it was more than easy to saddle her with the blame. Fair or not, the term "Spanish Influenza" became generally used.

There had been pandemics, epidemics of world-wide proportion, before. The fifty-year Plague of Justinian in the sixth century cost one hundred million lives, and the Black Death, which lasted through most of the fourteenth century, killed a quarter of the population of Europe. Influenza was not new either, with six major epidemics in the nineteenth century alone. The last, in the winter of 1889–90, affected over 40 percent of the world's population.

The big differences with the pandemic of 1918 were that it struck hardest at young adults, and that it was followed by a high incidence of pneumonia. It affected almost every populated area in the world and it is thought to have killed between twenty and twenty-two million people in just a few months. Assuming that not all deaths were reported, with doctors too busy and too exhausted to make reports; and given the fact that statistics-gathering was not then a sophisticated science; and, most important, that influenza had not until 1918 been considered a sufficiently serious disease (unlike typhoid, scarlet fever, and smallpox) to require that physicians report cases to their boards of health, that estimate may well be on the low side.

Other factors, too, could have affected the accuracy of the statistics. The onset of 'flu resembles a cold, so people who had a mild form of the disease may have believed they only had a cold. Conversely, it's reasonable to assume that in the midst of such a severe epidemic and with other diseases such as typhoid, diphtheria, scarlet fever, smallpox, and *Encephalitis lethargica* (sleeping sickness) prevalent around the same time, many deaths may have been wrongly attributed to influenza and the pneumonia which often followed.

The epidemic came in three major waves: the spring of 1918, the autumn of 1918, and the early months of 1919, with minor outbreaks occurring in various places through the 1920s. People who had been enjoying a mild fall trusted that the coming of cold winter weather would kill the germ; it didn't. Others blamed the cold, but in hot countries the death rate was every bit as high. India was reported to have suffered 12.5 million deaths. Weather had no bearing, it seemed, nor did attempts to keep away from outside contacts. Australia, which imposed a rigid quarantine, succeeded only in postponing the inevitable; influenza struck there in January 1919. During the first week of November, nearly fourteen thousand people died in England — more than twice the birth rate.

Ordinarily, respiratory disease strikes hardest at the very old and the very young; this time it was different. The primary target for this influenza epidemic was the young adult, making the onslaught particularly tragic both in personal terms and in terms of the strength of the country, coming as it did right on the heels of so many deaths in that same age group during the war. Although in some instances whole families succumbed to the disease, regardless of age, reports from across the country confirmed its deadly concentration on those in the prime of life. "Dangerous age 26–30," headlined the *Leader* in Regina, the *Vancouver Sun* reported that two-thirds of the victims were between twenty and forty, and in Ontario, of five hundred deaths reported to the vital statistics branch of the provincial board of health, 65 percent were of people between twenty and thirty years. One doctor noted that in any household he visited where there were three generations, he found the grandparents and the children doing well, and the parents very ill.

Spanish Influenza reached its height in Canada in the fall of 1918. It affected one in every six Canadians and killed between thirty thousand and fifty thousand; yet in the majority of history books it doesn't rate even a mention, and in others it is dismissed in a paragraph or two. Perhaps, as one writer suggested, compared with dying a glorious death defending your country, dying of 'flu was just not the way to go.

A Prince Edward Island woman, answering questions on a medical history form, said her mother had died in the influenza epidemic in 1918. "Oh, was there an epidemic then?" a young doctor asked casually. For her and the multitude of other Canadians whose lives were totally changed by this quixotic disease that orphaned numberless children, struck at random two families out of a whole block or all the members of a family except one, and for which there was no treatment and no cure, this was a major event ranking with wars and depressions.

'Flu Comes to Canada

Exactly when and where Spanish Influenza entered Canada, no-one is sure. The disease had made its appearance on this continent as early as March 11, 1918 when 107 American servicemen at Camp Funston, Fort Riley, Kansas sickened in one day. By the end of the training camp's five-week siege, 1,127 men had been stricken and 46 died of pneumonia following the 'flu.

In this country, however, troops who had been exposed to 'flu in Europe and who returned to Canadian ports in the late spring and early summer were almost certainly the major source of infection.

It was reported that among the men on the hospital ship *Araguaya*, which left England for Canada on June 26, 1918, there were servicemen already acutely ill with 'flu before they boarded the ship. During the voyage, from 23 to 40 percent of those sailing on her had the disease. The steamship *Somali*, sent back from Quebec City to the quarantine station at Grosse Isle because of 'flu on board, had 72 sick crew members within three days. The Med 1099 hospital ship landed at Halifax carrying 'flu and the *Nagoya*, with 100 sick men out of a total of 160 on board, landed at Montreal.

During the rest of the summer the disease seems to have lain quiet, but on September 8 the first major civilian outbreak occurred. At Victoriaville College, Quebec, 2 students came down with the disease, followed, alarmingly quickly, by 398 more. With no facilities at the college to deal with such an outbreak, boys well enough to travel were sent home across the province. Also in

September, 9 sailors from American ships died at Quebec City, and there was 'flu at the Polish Infantry Camp at Niagara, Ontario.

The scourge that was raging all over the world was well entrenched in eastern Canada, and it was carried rapidly across the country. Returning servicemen disembarking from crowded ships at Atlantic ports boarded trains that would take them home to cities, farms, and little towns from Newfoundland to British Columbia. Those who were not ill on landing were sometimes incubating the germ, and had to be taken off trains and hospitalized at cities across the country.

Dr. H.J.G. (Harold) Geggie was a junior medical officer at St-Jean, Quebec, the trans-shipment point where troops checked in. He was aghast at what he saw. Young men who had seemed perfectly well at night and had been on guard duty were dead by morning. It was a matter of hours.

Many times in later years he described to his son, Dr. Hans Geggie, what he considered to have been the most searing experience of his life. "My father couldn't get through to his senior officer the seriousness of the sickness. Having no proper facilities in this tiny sick bay, sometimes not even enough beds, he was in despair. Finally, frustrated beyond belief, he went over his superior's head and contacted influential people he knew at McGill University in Montreal rather than trying again and again to buck the military hierarchy." Within the week doctors and nurses arrived at St-Jean, as did a completely equipped hospital train, but Geggie says his father never forgot the suffering he saw, and the frustration he felt, knowing that while medical aid was within hailing distance it was so hard to reach.

During a welcoming ceremony for 922 returning troops de-training at Toronto in October, the men were asked about their voyage. "Oh, don't ask us about that," one replied. "We're just so glad to get home we want to forget about that part. . . . It was a disgrace to Canada to take men right out of hospitals and crowd us into that transport. We didn't have a bath or a change of clothing for over two weeks." His eyes filled with tears. "If that's all they think of us we don't need to expect much sympathy."

Between September 9 and December 12 there were a reported 10,506 cases of influenza among the 61,063 troops in Canada, and among the servicemen still overseas, there were 45,960 cases. One who caught the disease while overseas was W.E. Brown of the Fraser Valley in British Columbia. Not yet eighteen years old, he was serving as a gunner with the Royal Canadian Field Artillery, Forty-eighth Battery. Briefly behind the lines, the company was relishing the open farm-country atmosphere when Brown and two others were stricken with 'flu. There was no room for them in the advance hospitals so they lay on a grassy field with a groundsheet under them and a blanket on top. "I believe we recovered more quickly with that spartan treatment," he comments. Perhaps they did, because their illness lasted only three days.

Not only were troopships bringing 'flu to this country, they were also taking it back to Britain. Aboard the ships *City of Cairo*, the *Victoria*, and the *Huntsend*, sailing from Montreal and Quebec City, so many became ill that on their arrival in England the Canadian army had to segregate all its newly arrived fighting forces. A volunteer nurse at Reading, England remembered when an order was received to set up a new unit for 'flu cases. "By night we had moved into a converted convent. Almost before the desks were out the stretchers were in — 60 to 80 a classroom. We could hardly move between the cots. And, oh, they were so sick."

The *City of Cairo*, which sailed from Montreal on September 26 with a troopload of 1,057, reported 75 percent of all on board ill with influenza at some point during the voyage, and 32 deaths. On the *Huntsend*, also out of Montreal on that same day with 1,549 on board, 150 cases were seen by medical staff every day after the second morning out. Thirty-nine were buried at sea and one more died en route to hospital after landing. The *Victoria*, which sailed from Quebec on October 6 with a complement of 1,222, had 28 deaths during her passage.

The *Victoria*, built for South American coastal work, was not suitable for the cold weather of the North Atlantic. The ship was in Quebec harbor and had been cleared to join a convoy when influenza was discovered on board; a request was made for hospital accommodation ashore. "At this time the epidemic was at its height in Quebec, and every hospital and other building obtainable was full to the door with the sick. Absolutely no bed was available for many seriously ill cases in the City itself," said a report written on November 16, 1918 to the director general of medical services at Ottawa.

At the time the request for hospital accommodation ashore was made, there was in progress a storm so violent that it caused damage in the city and along the waterfront. Despite that, a medical officer did manage to get by tug from shore to the ship and, with the doctors on board, reached the conclusion that the sick men were generally feeling better. In any event, the report continued, "It is doubtful if any means could have been found for unloading them [the men] from the ship during the storm, and it would have been quite impossible to have brought the boat into the dock for this purpose."

The Victoria's thirty hospital beds and nine isolation beds were full even before the ship left port. Officers vacated their cabins to provide more accommodation for the sick men, and a "hospital" was improvised on the first troop deck. In all, during the twelve-day voyage to England, more than two hundred and fifty officers and men were ill with influenza and pneumonia. Twenty-eight died and were buried at sea with military honors, and when the Victoria arrived in England, 132 patients were taken to hospital.

Exhaustive inquiries were held into the problems on these troopships, and at least one medical officer was "given permission to retire both from the Service and the Militia." One ship's officer, who was named president of a court of inquiry into the deaths at sea, was recommended for special leave after the quarantine period in Britain had elapsed. He told his mother, in a very long letter from the camp in North Wales, that officers who had served at the front said that none of their previous experiences had been as harrowing as that voyage from Canada to Britain. After all the illness he had seen, and after sharing a cabin with an officer who died of 'flu, he was a thankful man to arrive safe and sound in Britain.

Similar problems were reported among United States troops. The American Journal of Public Health stated that mortality aboard troopships was twice that on land.

In fairness, authorities were faced with a tough dilemma. Fresh troops had to be taken to Europe to replace the wounded, dead, and returned fighting men; for safety, the ships travelled by convoy, making last-minute alterations to shipping dates to accommodate outbreaks of illness difficult, if not impossible.

Widespread Ravages of Spanish Influenza and Consequent Diseases

In Montreal Alone There Are 20,000 Cases of Influenza and From All Points Come News of Its Spread.—In Halifax We Have 500 Cases.

MONTREAL, October 13— It is estimated that there are nearly twenty thousand cases of grippe in Montreal and still more stringent regulations are enforced by the board of health to curb the epidemic. The order follows:

"All stores, shops, and bars of all kinds, retail and wholesale, except drug stores (for sale of drugs only) butchers' shops, grocery stores shall close at four o'clock.

"All churches, theatres, moving picture houses, dancing halls, billiard and pool rooms, bowling alleys, public baths, auction rooms, assembly or lecture halls shall remain closed.

"No athletics, sports, sporting gatherings of any kind or meetings open air or otherwise, where more than 25 people gather shall be allowed.

"All schools, public or private, including Sunday schools shall remain closed.

"Boarding schools shall not be allowed to receive day boarders or visitors and if allowed leave of absence pupils shall not be allowed to re-enter the school.

"Public offices including banks, government offices, municipal offices shall close not later than 4.30.

"All hospitals and dispensaries (except in urgent cases) shall be closed to all but emergency cases.

"No public shall be admitted to the courts except those essential to the prosecution of the cases called.

The board recommends most specially to the public not to crowd into any tramway and to avoid as much as possible any crowded train, tramway or railway station."

MONTREAL, October 13 — For spitting on the sidewalks twenty men appeared in court yesterday and were fined various amounts up to fifteen dollars or a month jail in each case.

OTTAWA, Oct. 13—It is estimated six hundred new cases of influenza developed here yesterday.

MONTREAL, October 13 — Of the 800 cases of influenza among soldiers in this district being treated there have been ninety-three deaths.

WINNIPEG, October 13—A proclamation practically suspends all public assemblies until all danger of infection from prevailing pulmonary disease is considered past. After Saturday night, all schools, theatres, churches, moving picture houses, business colleges, dance halls and other places where people assemble in numbers are to be closed and departmental and other stores, dining rooms, street

cars, railway trains, etc., are to be regulated under special precautionary measures. Municipalities which are practically suburban to Winnipeg, including Assinaboia, Transcona and Kildonan, and the city of St. Boniface, have adopted the same precautionary measures which extend to labor meetings and strike conferences. The area included in the above compromises the principal centres of population in Manitoba. In this area there will be no church services Sunday and special thanksgiving day services in churches.

TORONTO, October 13—Spanish influenza continues its steady advance thru every district of the city and province. The hospitals are practically all filled and the department of health in considering taking over some of the vacant hotel properties for additional hospital accommodation. Advertisements are in the press for voluntary workers as nurses, maids, orderlies cooks, etc., to strengthen the forces which are busily fighting the epidemic. Dr. Hastings has ordered all conventions and other large gathering to be postponed until epidemic abates. Among the conventions which will be cancelled are the Baptist convention of Ontario and Quebec, planned to open on Wednesday; the national association of electrical contractors and dealers, scheduled to start Monday; the three day conference of Loyal church workers "On Behalf of Israel" arranged for next week. The Ontario Sunday school convention has been planned for October 21. An order has been issued that only immediate relatives shall be allowed to attend funerals of persons who have died from influenza. To prevent the development of influenza in the wards of hospital for

children, visiting has been disallowed during the epidemic. The same course has been taken at the other hospitals.

TORONTO, October 13 — Toronto academy of medicine issued following appeal:

"In view of urgent demands for nurses to care for civilian and military sick and for hospital accommodation the council of the academy urges: "That all nurses who are at present not engaged in nursing, should report themselves for duty without delay to the central registry, to the lady superintendents of the hospitals, or to the medical authorities." At General hospital thirty nurses are suffering from influenza. One of them is Miss Hope Aylesworth, niece of Sir Aylesworth. Her condition is critical.

NEW YORK, October 13—The council of public health has made it a misdemeanor for any person to cough or sneeze in a public place anywhere in the state of New York without covering the mouth or nose. Violators will be rigidly prosecuted. The punishment will be $500 fine or one year in prison or both. It was decided to make influenza a reportable disease, which means that every case must be reported to the health officers by doctors, hotel proprietors, boarding house keepers and householders. Every new case will be placed immediately under state control From September 18 until today there have been 25,682 cases of influenza in New York city and 2,752 cases of pneumonia. Deaths from influenza numbered 1,052 and from pneumonia 1,509.

CAPETOWN, October 13—The worst plague that ever visited South Africa was nothing in comparison with the present epidemic of influenza. As a result of the epidemic there were 140 burials in Maitland cemetery today. The spread of influenza is diminishing in mining districts, where the hospital cases have been reduced from 20,000 to 3,000 since last week. Eight thousand cases have been reported at Durban. Some coal mines in Natal have been closed.

Five Hundred Cases Of Spanish Influenza Are Now in Halifax

HALIFAX, October 14—The fight against the spread of Spanish influenza by the city health board, continues unabated with encouraging results, compared with other Canadian cities, and shows daily that the precautionary measures taken in the early stages were fully

justified. While the disease had made considerable advance during the past week, it has not been nearly as alarming or disturbing as it would have been had not effective means been adopted by the health board, before the epidemic stage was reached. Prospects are still

Newspapers of the day carried alarming reports of the spread of the disease. (The Halifax Herald, October 14, 1918. Photo courtesy Public Archives of Nova Scotia)

Historically, epidemics travel along lines of communication and from east to west. That was true in Canada in that the first massive civilian outbreak took place in Quebec rather than in the west. Within weeks cases were appearing, almost simultaneously, right across the country. The troops, who were returning at the rate of thirty-four hundred per month after the signing of the armistice on November 11, carried some of the infection but by no means all. In Calgary, for instance, at the same time as a group of infected soldiers was taken from a troop train and isolated, a family newly arrived from New Brunswick, and the family of a man who had gone to New York to bring back his wife's body, were all found to have the disease. The movement of easterners to the west and back again in the summer and fall of 1918 in response to the call for forty thousand harvesters could not have helped matters either. A British Columbia woman remembers how unnerving it was. "We never knew where it would strike next," she said.

There was no central source of advice or control to deal with the emergency. Parliament had prorogued on May 24, 1918 and did not resume sitting until February 20, 1919. No federal health department existed. The Quarantine Service was administered by the Department of Agriculture from 1867 to 1918, and then by the Department of Immigration and Colonization. The Food and Drug Laboratory was located in the Department of Inland Revenue from 1894 to 1918, then briefly in the Department of Trade and Commerce. The formation of a new Department of Health was initiated in 1918, but it did not become fully operational until the following year.

The result of this widely disseminated responsibility was that decision-making in what was becoming an obvious emergency rested with provincial and municipal authorities, by no means all of them in agreement about what should be done. At first, many tried to soft-pedal the danger, perhaps feeling that panic would cause as much trouble as the disease. At the end of the first week in October, a spokesman for Ontario's provincial board of health still advised against closing schools and noted that children were less likely to infect one another in school than at home or on the playground. He recommended that health officers around the province consider the ordinary affairs of life. "They should not be moved from their duty by public clamor to adopt fussy and ill-advised measures which only serve to irritate the public and accomplish no useful purpose."

In Brantford, Ontario, Chairman T.J. Minnes of the board of health declared on October 5 that there was no need for alarm as the rumors were greatly exaggerated. On the same day a Brantford doctor died, and the hospital was too full to admit more cases. On October 9, the Toronto *Globe* said of Minnes: "He is able to state most emphatically, and is backed up by the most unquestionable authority, that there is no such thing existing in Brantford as Spanish influenza. There is no doubt that influenza or grippe is prevalent by far above the average for this season of the year, caused by the unreasonable climatic conditions at this time. He declares that there are 795 cases of grippe here, but not one is considered critical."

During the week of October 14, twenty-five hundred cases of 'flu were reported in Brantford, with ten deaths in one day, and on the sixteenth the *Globe* reported: "Dr. Pearson, Medical Officer of Health, declared that the situation was most serious, and people had to come forward and volunteer their services. So rushed has he been with private work that he has tendered his resignation as Medical Officer of Health, following upon friction in connection with the Board of Health, the Chairman of which, it is alleged, pooh-poohed all Dr. Pearson's requests, declaring that there was no Spanish influenza in the city, at a time when Dr. Pearson claimed there were over 100 cases."

As late as October 21 Saskatoon's medical health officer, Dr. Arthur Wilson, was quoted in the *Saskatoon Daily Star:* "This epidemic is nothing but the old form of influenza, or grippe. The only difference is that it has been given more publicity. At the last great outbreak which occurred in 1890, scarcely any publicity was given, and there were probably many more deaths at that time than there have been since this epidemic started."

A Toronto man threatened to cancel his subscription to his daily newspaper in protest at the grisly details being published. In New York State a Christian Scientist declared that the Chinese community where he lived remained largely unaffected because the people couldn't read the scary headlines, this comment despite the fact that during the month of October in New York City, 4,596 cases of 'flu were reported during one twenty-four hour period. By the end of the month the situation in that city was so desperate that a steam shovel had to be used to dig a trench in which to inter temporarily the bodies of influenza victims. At another cemetery, it was reported, four hundred bodies awaited burial.

The military, too, appeared to be concerned about keeping a low profile on the 'flu. On October 2 a message from the Department of Militia and Defence in Ottawa to the assistant director of medical services in Toronto stated it this way: "The disease, although extremely contagious, is not a serious one and every effort must be made to control alarm, not only among the troops but among the public and in the Press. The daily publication of statistics is very undesirable. The mortality is very low and due only to complications such as pneumonia. The period of illness is short and convalescence rapid."

But by October 9, the principal matron of Toronto's Military Base Hospital was sending urgent telegrams to civilian nurses around the province beseeching them to report for temporary duty; there were by then seventy cases of pneumonia in the hospital and an insufficient number of nursing sisters to care for them.

Dr. H.O. Howitt of Guelph, Ontario, said in a report to the Canadian Public Health Association on May 27, 1919: "The Government, for reasons of its own, did not make a statement as to the seriousness of the disease among the troops. . . . Never did the bulletins announce its presence quicker than modern conveyances could carry passengers."

On July 4, 1919, in a section on Canada, Britain's august medical journal the *Lancet* commented with an implied lift of the eyebrow: "It is scarcely understandable how medical officers simply waited for the inevitable."

The western provinces, having seen what their neighbors to the east were enduring, put up what defenses they could by refusing to allow trains to stop or by placing inspectors on board to give passengers a clean bill of health before they were allowed to de-train, and some instituted total quarantines. Feelings ran high on the subject. "You can fence your town and put out your men to stop the traffic on the roads, but YOU CAN'T DEFEAT THE PLAGUE THAT WAY," wrote A.F.A. Coyne in the *Edmonton Bulletin* on November 12. "It is in the air — and you can't fence that. While men and women are going down to death by the hundred, for God's sake and civilization, be British. TAKE YOUR CAR OUT NOW. DO YOUR DUTY TO YOUR CITIZEN NEIGHBOR IN DISTRESS. Your turn may be next to die. Die like a man fighting the battle for the sick."

Individual reactions ranged from fatalism to what one Saskatchewan woman described as "fear so thick that even a child could feel it." Coming after the losses so many had suffered in the war, for some there was only one way to deal with this new horror; they had to develop a shell over their emotions. "We were inured to sorrow"; "Every day there was someone we knew in the obituary columns"; "We got so we didn't even mourn." But if emotions were kept under control, compassion blossomed. In trouble as never before, the social barriers of the time were forgotten. Women who had never come closer to the mechanics of housekeeping than to instruct their cooks and chauffeurs, nursed people they didn't know, changed beds, cooked, and did laundry. The influenza epidemic cut across every stratum of Canadian life, affecting the rich as severely as it did the poor, and the just and the unjust suffered together.

Rumors were the order of the day. Stories circulated that Indians had been issued with unwashed blankets that had been used by infected troops. It was the cold; it was the unseasonable warmth; electricity was blamed; and, most of all, the enemy. A *Manitoba Free Press* editorial writer had this to say about the rumor that 'flu germs had been released by U-boat crews: "The Huns are sure handy people to blame anything on, but it is to be questioned whether one can blame them for everything that happens that does not seem just right."

The 'flu began, often, like a cold, with a cough and a stuffy nose, progressing to a dreadful ache that pervaded every joint and muscle, a fever that shot as high as 104 degrees, and a marked inclination to stay in bed. If it stopped there the patient was usually back to normal in a week, but when it developed into pneumonia the outlook was grave indeed. With no antibiotics to rely on, doctors could only turn to their time-honored cures, rest, liquids, and a lot of hope.

Pneumonia patients literally drowned in their own secretions. Dr. Herbert French, at a British military hospital, said he could be almost certain who was going to die judging just by the blue color of their faces. "It was when this dreaded heliotrope cyanosis appeared that one knew that the prognosis had now altered so completely that the patient was almost certain to die; a small percentage of cases managed to recover . . . but the great majority succumbed . . . it was amongst cases of this type that the great mortality of the epidemic occurred." About 40 percent of the people who developed pneumonia died.

Students in Dr. Margaret Patterson's Voluntary Aid Detachment course, under the auspices of St. John Ambulance, were warned: "Notice the color of your patient's lips and face. If there is not much air entering the lungs you will usually find that the lips become more or less purplish or dark blue instead of red, which shows the blood is not receiving the proper amount of oxygen." The purple-black skin was terrifying to everyone, but particularly so to people of central European descent who had been brought up on tales of the Black Death; many feared that this new disease was a reincarnation of the old plague.

One woman whose skin darkened felt she was so ill that she said one day to her sister, almost in surprise, "Well, I'm still here." "Yes, you are," her sister replied, "but you look awful, look at yourself in the mirror." They both laughed; it was true, she did look awful. Eva Mercer's skin had turned temporarily black. Her sister says: "I have never seen anything like it before or since, and when I told a doctor about it he was surprised to hear that she had recovered. My sister lived to be 87 years old!"

Delirium was commonplace. When schools closed in Saint John, New Brunswick, fourteen-year-old Lillian Clarke was kept close to home to avoid infection. One morning her mother was keeping her busy learning to make a dress with the treadle sewing machine. It seemed balky and uncooperative, sticking and tangling the thread. She was annoyed, too, by a mild ache in her back. "As the day went on I got more and more irritable and the machine more and more unco-operative. I now realize there was nothing wrong with the machine, rather my co-ordination was off."

About ten o'clock that night, after she had been asleep an hour, her parents heard shrieks from her bedroom. The ache in her back had been a precursor of 'flu, and now in her delirium she had vivid and terrifying dreams about elephants marching slowly past her bed. "Gradually they were going faster and faster and FASTER until I shrieked and woke up. I can still see the look between my parents and hear my father say: 'I'll get the doctor.' " Her chief memory of the two weeks that followed was the overwhelming desire to be left alone to rest. "To move a finger or even speak was too much exertion."

In Vancouver, Amy Biddle Dryer also suffered from fever-induced nightmares. Her dreams centered around the design of the quilt on her bed and left her with a lifelong aversion to the pattern. "To this day, a paisley pattern is obnoxious to me."

For some, the disease came on with no warning. Two Woodstock, Ontario, girls, working in the town of Paris, shared a room at the YWCA. One evening when the epidemic was at its height they attended a lecture together and then returned to their room. In the morning Claire Hunt Hunter called to her friend, "Vera, I'm going downstairs to breakfast." There was no reply, so she went ahead. After eating she went back upstairs to get her purse and called her roommate again. There was still no answer. "I pulled down the sheets. She was dead and cold. The doctor said she had died around two in the morning — the 'flu had got to her quick."

In Rivière Qui Barre, Alberta, Benjamin McKilvington was driving home by horse and buggy from a dance when he felt that a huge hand had squeezed his chest. The sensation passed, but by next morning he could not raise his head from the pillow. On the twenty-first day of his illness, he slept and dreamed. "I saw my mother, I could see the walls of the grave as I was going down, then all at once I saw my mother fall in and she passed me in that grave. I do not recall anything more, but that night I began to pick up and grow stronger." The dream was not precognitive; his mother lived a further ten years.

A doctor who called every day told the McKilvington family that a patient who had nosebleeds would recover more quickly and indeed, for Benjamin McKilvington's sister, that proved true. The hemorrhage she suffered filled a large white hand basin with blood, and a week later she was fine.

Benjamin's own recovery, on the other hand, was slow. It was twenty-one days before he could sit up on the edge of the bed, even with help, another twenty-one days before he could get dressed, and still another twenty-one before he could go outside. When at last he was able to get around he went to get weighed, supported by his mother on one side and his father on the other.

His normal weight was 137 pounds, but that day the scale showed
84 pounds. He wonders what the true figure was; at the time he
wore two suits of underwear, two top shirts, a sweater and a heavy
overcoat, huge mitts and mackinaw pants, two pairs of wool socks
under another very heavy pair, plus moccasins with insoles — and
a big fur cap.

There was no shortage of advice for the public and for doctors.
A gentleman in England contacted the high commissioner for
Canada, offering copies of a film he had produced and called "Dr.
Wise on Influenza," at a cost of fifteen pounds each. He explained
that the film started with a microscope view of millions of
microbes swarming like worms amid the blood corpuscles, and
that the story told ". . . how Brown took no precautions, neglected
obvious symptoms giving the disease as the result to others he
came in contact with and eventually succumbed to pneumonia
himself. His partner, however, acting on the advice of Dr. Wise,
avoided the disease in the manner shown. . . ." There is no record
of any sale for the film in Canada.

A vaccination program was tried. Since the discovery in
Germany in 1892 of Pfeiffer's bacillus, or *Bacillus influenzae*, it had
been generally believed that that organism was the cause of
influenza. Some scientists disagreed, and others thought it might
be only part of the cause. It seemed worthwhile, however, to
produce a vaccine made from these bacteria in the hope it would
be effective not only in immunizing the population, but also in
lessening the effects of the disease on those already sick.

These vaccines were produced by private laboratories and
provincial boards of health in Canada, and imported from the
United States. They were made available to civilian doctors, and
to military medical officers who administered them only to
servicemen who chose to have the shots. Chairman of Manitoba's
provincial board of health, Dr. Gordon Bell, announced that
anti-flu vaccine sufficient to treat everyone in Winnipeg had been
prepared, and from the Connaught Laboratories in Toronto came
word that they had produced a vaccine from eighteen strains of
dead influenza germs obtained from New York and Boston. Ten
thousand doses were distributed in Ontario, and on November 1
the *Montreal Star* reported: "Hurrying west on the transcontinental
trains today, thousands of small glass bottles containing anti-influenza serum are on their way from the Canadian Railway Board

to all railway centres in the west. Free inoculation will be offered all railway workers who desire the treatment as fast as the supply can be obtained. . . ."

Major F.T. Cadham of the Canadian Army Medical Corps in Winnipeg had been interested in vaccines since before the war, and when it became obvious that the epidemic was on its way he began work on a vaccine to combat it. He reported to the *Canadian Medical Association Journal* the results of inoculations given on a voluntary basis to 4,842 of the 7,600 soldiers in the area. "From October 1st, 1918, to February 28th, 1919, five hundred and twenty soldiers were admitted to this hospital suffering from the disease. . . . Among two hundred and eighty-two inoculated seventeen developed pneumonia and five died. Of the five that died, three had received their first inoculation on the day they were admitted to the hospital. One developed the disease three days subsequent to the first inoculation and one ten days subsequent. The latter soldier was suffering from tubercular glands of the neck. No soldier died who had been admitted subsequent to his second inoculation. Among the two hundred and thirty-eight admitted who had not been inoculated with the vaccine there occurred forty cases of pneumonia and seventeen deaths."

An indication of the panic and the hope among the general population was that Dr. Cadham had to have a police escort as he drove from his home to his office, so anxious were people to get the vaccine.

Representatives of Quebec's Superior Board of Health travelled to Boston to appraise the value of the vaccines in use in Massachusetts. Later, when vaccines were offered to Quebec by Connaught Laboratories, the board elected not to distribute them in Quebec on the grounds that the vaccines were still at the experimental stage and none had been recognized as scientifically effective against the disease. Instead, they recommended that the public rely on their physicians' advice as to the best treatment.

No-one was sure of the value of the vaccines. Dr. J.J. Heagerty, bacteriologist and assistant medical officer at the Grosse Isle Quarantine Station, said later in the *Canadian Medical Association Journal*: "Unfortunately for the health officer and the practitioner, there were a number of vaccines on the market during the recent epidemic. All of them had their advocates; all of them their detractors. . . . Between them all, the practitioner was lost in a sea of confusion, was doubtful of all of them, used them, if at all, with trepidation, and then only as a last resort in hopeless cases, never as a preventive. The health officer was equally confused, did not feel that he was justified in instituting measures for general vaccination, and meanwhile the disease spread."

Dr. Victor C. Vaughan, acting surgeon general of the United States army, summed up the feelings of a lot of doctors: "I say that in the face of the greatest pestilence that ever struck this country,

Enterprising pharmacists were soon advertising the new vaccines. (The Leader, Regina, Saskatchewan, October 31, 1918. Photo courtesy Saskatchewan Archives Board)

we are just as ignorant as the Florentines were with the plague described in history," and the chief medical officer of the local government board of England, Sir Arthur Newsholme, said: "I know of no public health measures which can resist the progress of pandemic influenza."

Confusion and bewilderment reigned. Still, in the light of the medical knowledge of the times, the vaccines developed were a commendable attempt at controlling the ravages of the epidemic; not until the 1930s would the true cause of the influenza of 1918 be known.*

---

*See Chapter 7, "And in Its Wake."

East to West
North to South
Everywhere Is 'Flu

THE ATLANTIC SEABOARD

At the city of St. John's, the easternmost tip of the continent and capital of the then Dominion of Newfoundland, a ship arrived in port on September 30, 1918, carrying three sailors sick with 'flu. They were taken to hospital and reported by the St. John's *Daily News* on October 3 to be seriously ill. The following day an American vessel that landed at Burin also had on board three sick crew members, and hasty arrangements were made to take them by train to hospital in St. John's. "The only notice the Health Department had of their coming was a message from the magistrate at Placentia stating he had heard they were on the train," reported the newspaper.

The first local cases of influenza were only two days in appearing. On the fourteenth of October the acting medical officer of health announced the closing of schools, theatres, moving picture houses, and concert halls; some of them seized the opportunity to renovate their premises. The King George V Institute on Water Street, popularly known as the Seamen's Institute, was taken over for temporary hospital use, and W.S. Halfyard, colonial secretary, proclaimed in the *Royal Gazette*

Extraordinary that all vessels entering any Newfoundland port would be placed under quarantine until pronounced free of infection.

The Empire Steam Laundry on King's Road notified its customers: "Owing to the greater part of our staff being ill, we are not able to accept any work for delivery this week."

Eight deaths in the space of twenty-four hours, all young adults, were reported in the city on October 26. Churches were still closed on Armistice Day, a time when many people would like to have been able to go to church, but they reopened a week later and by mid-December the emergency in the city seemed to be past.

This encouraging situation did not prevail in outlying areas. Reports of 'flu continued to come in from Lark Harbour, New Melbourne, Exploits, Fortune Harbour, and Broom Bottom. Word came from Middlebrook and Gambo that they were trying desperately to cope with two hundred sick people. The *Harbour Grace Standard* printed funeral notices for each person who died on sheets of twelve-by-eighteen-inch paper edged in deep black, and posted them throughout the town. While Harbour Grace schools were closed and most public meetings discouraged, church services were allowed to continue.

There were two hundred cases at Indian Islands, and every home at New Pelican was affected. From Green's Harbour on New Year's Day, 1919, the Reverend Robert Smith wrote: "Whatever it is grips the heart dreadfully and it needs stimulant. If you (I mean the Dept. of course) cannot send two doctors for the place, please try to send medicines. If I could get my orders filled immediately I would try to battle on." The deputy colonial secretary responded two days later with the word that one parcel of medicines had been sent, and another would follow. Mr. Smith wrote on January 9 to say that the immediate need for a nurse had passed, adding that he was too tired to write more than necessary. "I was out nearly all last night after being down the shore nearly all day and I've been very busy here today."

Along the Labrador coast the Grenfell Mission and, farther north, the Moravian Mission, were actively engaged in both spiritual and practical aid for the people. After the ice formed in the fall, and until the water was clear enough in June for supply and mail boats to navigate, the whole coast was cut off from communication with St. John's.

To this quiet world, unfortunately still accessible by ship that fall, the 'flu came to work its fury. It came first to Cartwright at Sandwich Bay, via the mail boat *Sagona* on October 20; four of the crew were ill, and two days after the ship had left most of the settlement was sick. The boat continued to work its way north, leaving the germ at every community it visited.

Cartwright was a considerable settlement; the one hundred residents eked out a living hunting and fishing. The Hudson's Bay post consisted of fourteen or fifteen buildings, including the Big House, which was the home of the manager and his family, and the various stores, offices, and warehouses.

One of the clerk-apprentices, fourteen-year-old Bert Swaffield, son of the retired factor, had stayed on to work for his father's successor, Hayward Parsons; it was the beginning of what was to be a forty-six-year career with the company. Part of his job was to help check off cargo from the ships which arrived frequently from St. John's during the summer months. It was a task that normally took ten to twelve hours and was overseen by the ship's purser. On that October 20 arrival, because of the sick crewmen, Bert also helped with the moving of the supplies onto the dock, and altogether the work took two or three days. That first night, when he went up to the Big House where he took his meals, he found the purser lying on the sofa in the front room, too ill to take responsibility for the cargo he had delivered.

Hayward Parsons was the first in the community to catch the disease, followed not long after by Bert Swaffield. "Although I was sick for a month, I was one of the lucky ones," he remembers. "Many of those who got it later also got pneumonia."

Along with the mail and shipments of clothing, lumber, fuel oil, and groceries, the SS *Sagona* had brought both the influenza and, via newspaper reports, the residents' first inkling of its existence.

The Reverend Henry Gordon of the Grenfell Mission had been away on a short sea tour of the area. When he returned to his Cartwright base on the morning of October 30, this chilling scene met his eyes: "Not a soul to be seen anywhere, and a strange, unusual silence. Going along the path to the parsonage, we met one of the Hudson's Bay Company men staggering about like a

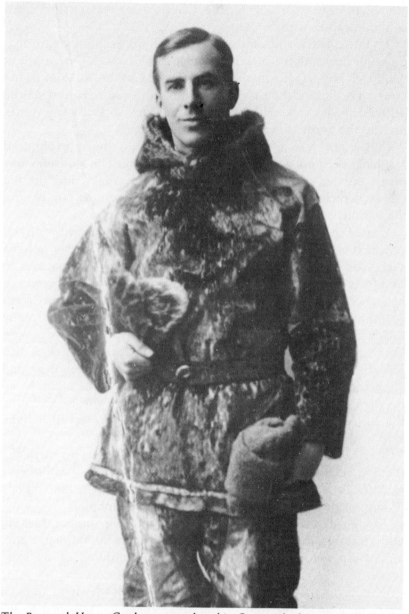

The Reverend Henry Gordon returned to his Cartwright base in Labrador on October 30, 1918 to find the community stricken with influenza. His diary recorded the devastating impact of the epidemic, in which one-quarter of the small village's population was wiped out. (Photo courtesy Provincial Archives of Newfoundland and Labrador)

drunken man, and from him learnt the news that the whole settlement was prostrated with sickness. It has struck the place like a cyclone, two days after the Mail boat had left. After dinner I went on a tour of inspection among the houses, and was simply appalled at what I found. Whole households lay inanimate all over their kitchen floors, unable to even feed themselves or look after the fire. No-one complained of any particular pain, a bad headache and an utter exhaustion seemed to be the prevalent symptoms. . . . I think there were just four persons in the place who were sound. . . . A feeling of intense resentment at the callousness of the authorities, who sent us the disease by the Mail-boat, and then left us to sink or swim, filled one's heart almost to the exclusion of all else. The helplessness of the poor people was what struck to the heart. The one and only Doctor on the coast (Dr. Paddon of the International Grenfell Association) was one hundred and eighty miles away, and might have been ten thousand for what chance he could have of getting his assistance to us."

Gordon wrote in his journal for Friday, November 1: "The weather is getting bitterly cold. . . . Very few of our people have any stock of Firewood home, and scarcely a house with any sawed up. Roly [Bird, Gordon's assistant] and I set to work and sawed and split as hard as we could go. . . . Mrs. Parsons, the wife of the new agent of the HBC [Hudson's Bay Company], who has been a trained nurse, is of tremendous assistance. She gets about among the sick and, with the few drugs at her disposal, does wonders. My head is beginning to get heavy. I hope against hope that I may be able to keep fit."

Saturday, November 2: "Feeling rotten, head like a bladder full of wind. Felt able to get up, however. . . . About noon, I received word that young Howard Fequet had died. . . . Digging graves in the Cartwright cemetery is labour out of the ordinary. Good folk many years ago chose the spot, evidently for its prominence, quite forgetful of the fact that a prominent spot in this country means a nut that the glacier or the sea was not able to crack. About one foot of soil lies over the ground, then comes a layer of tightly compressed blackish gravel, which reminds me of nothing so much as the carbon that accumulates on the cylinder of a motor engine. Beneath this are huge boulders almost cemented in with the pressure. When, in addition to all these other difficulties, the ground is frozen, it may be imagined what the work entails."

Tuesday, November 5: "Felt very sick. I know Mr. Parsons came to ask me about burying somebody or other. I thought it was myself at the time."

Gordon struggled on and gradually regained the strength he needed. The last mail boat of the season, the SS *Seal*, arrived on November 7, and all who were strong enough turned out to help in the unloading of freight. Gordon was concerned about the fate of communities surrounding Cartwright, but there was little anyone could do because the weather was too stormy to go out in boats. Swaffield recovered at last and set to work making coffins. "We could hardly keep up," he remembers. "Someone died almost every day." Also, he accompanied Mrs. Parsons, who was pregnant at the time, on her rounds among the houses, carrying her meagre stock of medications — aspirin, liniment, and poultices. "It was very upsetting, people crying, children dying everywhere."

By the end of November, twenty-six people out of the one hundred residents of Cartwright had died.

News came finally from one nearby settlement. At North River, out of twenty-one people, ten had died and still lay in their beds; no-one had the strength to bury them. The weather had calmed a little, and a party of five from Cartwright, one of them Henry Gordon, fought their way through the treacherous new ice to North River. They dug a huge pit for the bodies, rolled them in their bedclothes, and laid them in the mass grave. One survivor, a woman of seventy-two years who had been a midwife for the community and had delivered Bert Swaffield, as well as the other children of the Hudson's Bay families, had lived all alone for the nine days since the last of her family had died. She had been without a fire and with almost no food. From buckets of solid ice she chopped fragments with an axe and thawed them in a cup under her arms, while outside the starving dogs tore at the door.

In December, as the rescue party travelled along the coast, they encountered a few settlements where the sickness had not penetrated but news of it had. "We had grown so used to death that we had almost lost all sentiment about it," Gordon wrote. "Some of the settlements up the bay had miraculously escaped the sickness, and the people were really afraid of us. Of course, we never tried to enter any of these places, but it seemed strange to see anyone we happened to meet out on the ice 'convey themselves away from us.' "

At Mountaineer Cove, where once four families had lived, the group found only the pitiful remains of one. Five little children, all that were left, were getting along on their own in a house where four had died and still lay. Gordon made arrangements for neighbors to take the children in until he could contact relatives. From North River came more bad news: three more had died.

When, late in November, presumably from the captain of the last mail boat, the SS *Seal*, the offices of the Hudson's Bay Company in St. John's got word of the dire straits of the Labrador people, they requested that a steamer be sent with medical stores and aid. A disappointing response came from the colonial government: "A meeting of the Executive Government was convened, and the question was given earnest consideration. Efforts were then made to procure a steamer . . . it was found, however, that there were no coal supplies at Battle Harbor, and the ships did not have sufficient coal to enable them to go so far north as Sandwich Bay, and under these circumstances the two vessels in question could not proceed. It was practically impossible to get any other ship, for the owners would want a guarantee of payment should the ship be hampered by ice and kept there for the winter, while the Government would also have to stand the cost of special insurance.

"It is thought too that as the date of the letter from Cartwright was the 8th, and now three weeks have passed, the epidemic would be waning, and by the time a ship from St. John's reached there it would probably be all over. In view of the above circumstances, the Government regret that it was impossible to do anything in connection with the sending of a ship."

Their judgment was wrong; the emergency was far from over.

Farther up the coast, at Okak, a man and his wife and two of their children died, leaving only an eight-year-old girl. By some miracle she survived five weeks alone. The Reverend Walter Perrett, superintendent of the Moravian Mission, described her ordeal: "The huskies (dogs) now began to eat the dead bodies, and the child was a spectator of this horrible incident. So mad did the beasts become, upon tasting human flesh, that they attacked the child herself, biting her arm. How she escaped being devoured alive is described by the surviving natives as a miracle — which it undoubtedly was." It was thirty degrees below zero. The little girl had used the last of the Christmas candles to melt snow for drinking water.

The people of Okak had been warned that disaster would befall them. Emelia Merkuratsuk explained: "The sign was the Northern Lights were bright red. Even the snow was pink from the reflection. Then we knew there was going to be something happening which we never thought would be anything so bad as epidemic flu."

The Eskimos followed a pattern of travel by boat in the fall, before freeze-up, settling themselves in outlying areas for a winter of fishing and seal hunting. Once the ice was strong, they could move about at will. At the hunting grounds, Emelia's husband and two children died and another woman, whose family had all died too, shared Emelia's house because there were fewer bodies there. At night the two women looked out at an unusually large star moving westward and wondered what it was. They didn't know the date but realized from the full moon that it must be nearing Christmas. Most of the people died, and at last those who were left made their way back to Okak. There they found only three men and a few women and children still living. Mr. Perrett described the task undertaken by the men: "The ground was frozen as hard as iron, and the work of digging was as hard as ever work was. It took about two weeks to do it, and when it was finished it was 32 feet long, 10 feet wide, and 8 feet deep. Now began the task of dragging the corpses to the pit. They laid 114 bodies in the pit, each wrapped in calico, sprinkled disinfectants over them, and covered the trench, placing rocks on top to prevent the dogs from tearing it up."

When she was seventy-nine years old, Emelia Merkuratsuk looked back on the winter of 1918. "There were many belongings and clothing lying around outdoors. Even now I don't like to see clothing lying around outdoors. Also I don't like to see people sleeping on the floor. Those things are reminders of the horrible sickness that once happened when I was still in my young life."

At Hebron, just about the time the people were due to begin their autumn migration, the Moravian Mission boat *Harmony* arrived in port. Although the missionaries, advised by the captain that there was 'flu in Newfoundland, cautioned the native people to avoid contact with the sailors, many of them were too excited to heed the warning and clambered aboard the ship. When the *Harmony* left, it towed some of the Eskimo boats toward the fishing areas. The people set up camp and began to place their nets, but they were already beginning to sicken. Those who were strong enough made the arduous journey back to Hebron, pulling by oar against heavy seas. At Hebron thirteen-year-old Joshua Obed, sick with 'flu, lay beside another sick man. "All of a sudden he started to lean up against the wall and then he fell dead on the pillow. My brother, even though he was sick, dragged that dead man to the door."

It was the custom to hold Single Men's Day on January 25 for unmarried men and boys over thirteen. Joshua Obed said: "I never had my day 'cause the sickness came, besides that I was the only single man left in Hebron. ... After a while nobody else died, and we were the only ones left in the whole community. Before they died, people had dark spots on the insides of their hands and lips."

Bodies at Hebron were consigned to the water. Men cut holes in the ice and, weighting the bodies with rocks, dropped them through. Joshua Obed remembered one body that would not sink despite the rocks and two brand-new anchors on the end of the rope. "His name was Nathaniel and before he died he said he didn't want to be buried in the water." An eerie funeral service, conducted in a fierce wind and blinding blizzard at thirty degrees below zero, saw those people laid to their rest.

The stark total was reported by Mr. Perrett: "Out of a population of 220 at Hebron only 70 remain. Of Okak's 266 only 59 remain."

On January 9, 1919, the first good news in many weeks came via a Labrador man who, discharged from the army, had made his way up the coast on foot. He brought word that the war had ended. So cut off from the outside world was the coast of Labrador that it had taken two full months for this momentous news to reach them.

During all of that appalling winter, the missionaries worked night and day to care for the sick people, to give them spiritual consolation, and finally to dig graves for those who did not survive.

For Henry Gordon, at Cartwright, an urgent priority was to protect the mass graves against predatory animals. He arranged to have the graves strongly fenced with wire, knowing that wood could not survive the climatic conditions of successive winters. He wrote a report to the colonial secretary, explaining at length the conditions the people had faced and the steps he had taken in regard to fencing the graves.

The government's response, the following June, was to dispatch the SS *Terra Nova* to Labrador, carrying a doctor and a stock of medicines, and an expert carpenter with a quantity of prepared lumber "so that coffins may be made for the proper burial of those who died last fall and winter and were buried in the best manner possible."

In view of this gesture, seven months after the event, Gordon's reply was restrained. Part of it reads: "I am exceedingly sorry that such a step should have been taken without some communication having been made with myself on the matter, for I could have saved the Government the expense and (please forgive me) the rather ridiculous situation of the man who came to shut the stable door after the horse was stolen!"

Dr. Wilfred Grenfell, beloved by all in Labrador, was a practical man who once, when the mail steamer arrived in the midst of a church service, postponed the rest of the sermon after intoning: "Dear Lord, we know that we have You always with us. However, we rarely see the mail steamer. Please excuse us; we will be back shortly." His reaction was couched in blunter terms than Gordon's: "The intolerable insult of sending down at the expense of the Government a doctor, an undertaker, a policeman, and fifteen hundred feet of lumber (with provision for their own personal comfort and safety of a nature which, with your sense of humor, I leave you to surmise), really made the people nearly throw them in the sea when they landed, after they had refused to send help when it was needed. I do not think that those who are now your colleagues could possibly have had any imagination. I do not suggest that they had no heart." He closed with the pointed statement: "Personally I congratulate the country on your having assumed the position of Colonial Secretary."

Thirty-five years later, the then governor of Newfoundland wrote: "It was only many weeks after the scourge had done its worst that the news of the trouble came through to St. John's. The Government at once considered what could be done, but at that time of year it was felt that any relief expedition would have involved grave risk to the lives that carried it, with the certain knowledge that it was too late to arrest the plague. The lesson to those responsible for administration was a bitter one."

At a conservative estimate, more than one-third of the people of the Labrador coast perished in the 'flu epidemic during the winter of 1918-19.

THE MARITIME PROVINCES

By the fall of 1918, the city of Halifax, Nova Scotia still had not fully recovered from the December 6, 1917 explosion when a Norwegian freighter carrying supplies for Belgian relief collided in the harbor with a French ship loaded with munitions. In the resulting explosion 1,630 people were killed, and 9,000 injured. The following day, as people struggled to find missing relatives and friends amid the wreckage, a severe blizzard blew up, adding to the problem of shelter for this city where six thousand homes had been destroyed and twelve thousand damaged. Schools did not reopen until March.

Among the many to aid Halifax were the people of Massachusetts, who sent workers, medical personnel, and $150,000 worth of supplies. Haligonians did not forget, and when the 'flu epidemic struck Massachusetts in 1918, they sent nurses to help. Two who went were sisters, Winnifred and Georgena Flemming of Londonderry. The epidemic struck on September 7 at Camp Devens, near Boston, where 45,000 men were being trained for the war overseas. In their midst was one man suffering from influenza and in just over two weeks, 12,500 men had the disease. By the end of September, 780 had died.

Before long, Nova Scotia needed all its nurses at home. By early October the epidemic was raging in Sydney and Halifax, and on October 9 an ad appeared in the Halifax *Morning Chronicle:* "Nurses! Nurses whose services will be available to undertake the care of epidemic Spanish Influenza in Nova Scotia please register." All public gatherings were prohibited, and an attempt was made to placard those houses where 'flu existed. The attempt was unsuccessful for the most part, because people were reluctant to admit contagion.

With captains, engineers, and mates stricken with the disease, the ferry between Halifax and her sister city Dartmouth operated with great difficulty. The waiting room was small, and to keep infection down a regulation was passed that not more than ten people should occupy it at one time.

Hugh Mills, now chairman of Mills Brothers department store, was twenty when the 'flu struck Halifax. "Times were hard in those early days, and we took in boarders. Luckily, one of them was an army doctor." Mills got 'flu the day after Christmas. He recovered in about a week and although he was left weak and tired, he continued with his plan to open a small store — the same one that now employs more than one hundred people.

In Halifax and Dartmouth, public gatherings were forbidden until November 6.

Along the south coast of Nova Scotia, at Boutilier's Point, most residents worked for one large company and bought their food and clothing from the company store. Ralph Boutilier, who was twelve then, remembers that wages were so low that most people owed the company money. When payday came the company kept the cheque and gave the employee a receipt, leaving him still in debt. For the Boutilier family of seven, wood to keep the old drum stove going was the most pressing need. The father went to cut wood, wearing shoes that were not watertight; as long as the ground was frozen hard he was all right, but on one mild day his feet got damp. He tied brush around them to protect them as well as he could, but got frostbite that kept him home for a long period. It was a hard time.

The epidemic was bad in the Boutilier's Point area around Christmas time, a great disappointment to the children who had looked forward to a Christmas celebration with a concert planned by the teacher. But by Christmas time, those children who didn't already have influenza were coming down with it. "Nobody could even whisper, let alone sing. That was the end of our merry Christmas," Boutilier remembers. The doctor, who lived eight miles away, made his calls to the village by horse and sleigh, warmly dressed in a fur coat and cap. Very few people had money to pay him but he came anyway, tending faithfully to his patients. Sadly, this beloved doctor got 'flu himself and died./

At Mahone Bay the Zwicker family, descendants of 1750s settlers, lived in a comfortable frame house with a kitchen range and a small living-room stove, neither of which was ever allowed to go out in winter. One night during the epidemic Mrs. Zwicker wakened and called out for water. Effie Zwicker Matchett, then sixteen, brought a cup of water, but her mother asked for more. "Bring me the whole dipperful," she said. "I'm so hot." When she had drunk it all she was a little better and went back to sleep. In the morning she still felt somewhat draggy, so the doctor was called. "You've had the 'flu, but you're over it," he told her. He placarded the house and told Effie she could go out because she couldn't carry the disease, but no-one could enter. However, when her father, a timekeeper for a lumber company, came home a few days later and was met with the news that he couldn't enter, he ignored the ruling.

All the churches, schools, and moving picture houses in the town were closed. Infected homes were placarded with signs reading "Spanish Influenza" in large black print.

Vivian Read Allen was just entering her teens when 'flu came to her home at Upper Nappan. Although cash was scarce, the Reads were prosperous farmers. In 1916 they had bought a Chalmers nine-seat passenger car accommodating four in the back, two in the little side seats, and three in front. It wasn't used in winter; people got around then by horse and sleigh. They had a telephone too, number 906, ring 5, and they got news from the weekly Amherst *News & Sentinel*. Their house was a wooden Cape Cod style, with a hall through the centre, a living and dining room on one side, and kitchen, pantry, and scullery on the other.

Out of the Read family of sixteen children, only the mother and one child escaped the 'flu in the winter of 1918. "My father and mother had planned to go into Amherst a few days before Christmas to do the holiday shopping, but before they could get away my father became ill and had to go to bed. There were no Christmas gifts that year, and no tree, but we were too sick to care." Each day two more children became ill. On Christmas Day, when the doctor came to call, he counted noses; there were eight patients in bed.

One of the biggest chores for Mrs. Read, who said afterward that she hadn't had time to bother getting sick — "fortunately for us," her daughter says — was the daily laundry. It was done in a big round tub that sat on springs and had a handle to be swung back and forth, a scrub board, and a wringer. Between non-stop washings, she bathed the patients and put poultices on their chests.

Those were the days of great neighborliness. The Reads had one hundred cattle, including twelve cows, and twelve horses in the barns. No-one in the family was well enough to look after the animals, so friends and neighbors took over. "They were afraid to come into the house so they delivered the milk to the doorstep and my young brother, the only one of the children to escape 'flu, carried it in."

No part of Nova Scotia escaped the scourge. Cape Breton's Marble Mountain was so overrun with 'flu that it was likened to "a deserted village."

At Caledonia, in about mid-November, influenza was brought home to the De Long family by one of the boys, who had helped care for a fellow worker at a lumber camp. He caught the disease himself, and at home the four younger children in the family got it too. Their parents made a bed in the kitchen where they snatched naps whenever they could, between bathing the children and plying them with drinks of water to get their fevers down. Neighbors were afraid to enter the house but they took away and returned laundry, and left cooked dinners outside. It was nearly Christmas by the time the children were allowed out of bed. Leona De Long Baker, who was then thirteen, remembers the good doctor's answer when her brother asked if he could eat some baked beans for Christmas dinner. "Just one," the doctor told him, holding up one finger warningly.

Mary Oickle Kaulback, then living at Victory, Annapolis County, was four years old. "My mother, father, brother and sister and I all had it at the same time and I remember us all in bed at once with a practical nurse in attendance. We all survived except my mother, who was pregnant and died in childbirth.

"My uncle also died in that epidemic and I remember the long black hearse drawn by two black horses, and the driver with the tall black hat. No other family in the village was affected as we were."

Nineteen eighteen was a bad year on Prince Edward Island, with the early months notable for "extreme inclemency and continuous stormy weather," according to the reports of school inspectors. "All through the months of January, February and March, storm succeeded storm. So banked were the roads and so severe was the cold that it was well nigh impossible for even grown-up people to travel, much less school children."

In the spring, with so many farm laborers away at war, the department of education reintroduced the old system of spring and fall vacations. The move relieved the labor shortage but put the school year even farther behind. "And thus it was that the first half of the school year passed — unfavorable conditions and interruptions retarding progress right along."

Then came the 'flu. Again, schools closed all over the island. By October 16 there were six hundred and fifty cases in Charlotte-town and public funerals were forbidden.

The Cullen family, whose farm was part of what is now the airport at Charlottetown, was working toward a traditional double celebration: the completion of the harvest and the November 9 birthday of the head of the family, Timothy Cullen, which was marked every year by a big chicken dinner with all the trimmings. It was not to be, that year or ever again.

The Cullens had been careful to stay away from the city and infection, but the time came when Timothy and his two sons had to leave the farm to load potatoes and turnips on a Nova Scotia schooner. Two of the ship's crew were ill, and within a few days the boys who had been in contact with them had influenza. Mrs. Frances Landrigan Cullen (called Fanny), one daughter, and two younger sons were next.

Another daughter, Ellen Mary, was at university in Antigonish. She too had 'flu and couldn't help. Cecilia Cullen De Lory, not yet seventeen, was teaching in a one-roomed school at East Royalty, and when the school closed she came home. She and her father settled the patients into two large rooms downstairs with a fireplace in each, and in an upstairs bedroom where there was a coal stove. A cousin, aged nineteen, kept the big kitchen range going to heat the house and to warm bricks for the patients' beds. The doctor came every day from Charlottetown, and Cecilia and her father gave the patients strengthening sips of whisky, brandy, or rum in water, and rubbed their chests with camphorated oil.

On November 1, Fanny Cullen's 'flu changed to pneumonia and nine days later, on the tenth, she died. She was forty years old. By then the churches had reopened, and a funeral service was held for her next day at St. Dunstan's Cathedral. Timothy Cullen never again allowed any marking of his birthday.

Travellers sickened in hotels everywhere. A Prince Edward Island member of parliament, staying at a large Ottawa hotel, was sick alone for three days before someone checked and got help for him.

Captain John Read, master of *The Prince Edward Island*, the first car ferry between Borden, Prince Edward Island, and Cape Tormentine in New Brunswick, became ill with 'flu during the night. He took hot lemonade, quinine, and aspirin and after perspiring profusely all during the night hours in his cabin, in the morning he called the quartermaster to bring him dry clothing and buckets of sea water. He sloshed the icy salt water over himself, dried off, and dressed — and took the ferry out as usual.

Captain Read's daughter, Georgie Read Barton, now a prominent artist, was sixteen. She took a walk along the shore one morning, feeling fine: "But when I came back I wasn't feeling just right so my mother took my temperature. It was 101 degrees. In an hour, 102, then 103, and 104." Her fourteen-year-old sister, the only one in the family to escape the malady, took over the care of the rest of the family, making boiled onion poultices for their chests and big pots of soup to strengthen them. People were afraid to come any closer to the house than the end of the lane, about two hundred yards away, where they left groceries. On a night when temperatures flared very high, the doctor in Summerside sent medicine by horse and sleigh; Captain Read met the messenger at Bedeque, the halfway point, to bring it home to his family at Borden.

Across the island that fall there were 101 deaths: there was one on the last day of September, the graph peaked in October with 51 deaths, there were 28 in November, and 21 in December.

A ship of the Seagull Patrol attached to the British North West Atlantic Squadron, HMCS *Festubert*, passed Brier Island off the west coast of Nova Scotia and set a course for Saint John, New Brunswick. Ordinary Seaman George A. Davies of Belfast, Prince

Edward Island, had a two-hour duty at the wheel from midnight, after which he was scheduled to take the watch on the bridge. At two o'clock in the morning, in preparation for the Atlantic winds and spray, he added to his regular naval uniform a parka outfit half an inch thick and a set of oilskins on top of that. When he was ready to leave the chartroom, the first officer appeared, looking white and miserable. "You'll have to take over my watch," he told Davies. "I'm so sick I can't hold up my head any longer."

By the time the *Festubert* docked at Saint John, every officer aboard, including the captain, had been stricken with 'flu. Three of them were so severely ill that they had to be taken to hospital; yet not one of the crew got the disease. There was no explanation.

Davies, then nineteen years old, was given leave. He has never forgotten the gloom of Saint John that winter day; it seemed every second house had a black rosette on the door. He asked what it meant and was told that someone in each of those houses had died of Spanish Influenza.

When Christine Ryan Fewings answered the door of her home in Saint John one morning, it was to hear sad news: a family friend, the mother of several children, had died of 'flu. As she talked with the messenger, the telephone rang; it was word that another friend had died. She went to see what she could do. "As I entered the house I could see how ill the grandmother was. The wee tot was clinging to her apron as she tried desperately to get some liquid food ready. Both the parents died of pneumonia that day." She was able to contact the St. James Street Salvation Army hostel, which took care of the grandmother, and family members took the baby to raise.

When several of the eight Murphy children at Tabusintak caught 'flu, neighbors helped out. Helen Murphy Robertson, who was thirteen, says: "Everyone raised enough beef, pork and chicken, and had salted or smoked fish and lots of vegetables in the cellar, enough to see us through the winter. But we needed flour and molasses and beans, and the neighbors brought those." One of the elder brothers of the family, who worked away from home, came night and morning to feed the horse and cows, and to carry wood and water to the back door.

REGISTER

— OF —

Attendance, Grades of Instruction, and General Standing

OF THE PUPILS ATTENDING SCHOOL

— IN —

Grades 4 & 5.

~~District No.~~ *7*   Parish of   *Newcastle*   County of *Northumberland*

Town of Newcastle

WITH A RECORD OF VISITATION

Closed for Flu Oct. 10th — Nov. 25th — 1918
" by Board of Health Dec. 16 — Dec. 20th 1918

PRESCRIBED BY THE BOARD OF EDUCATION FOR THE SCHOOLS OF NEW BRUNSWICK

PUBLISHED FOR THE EDUCATION DEPARTMENT

FREDERICTON, N.B.

1918

During the height of the epidemic, it was necessary to close schools temporarily. This school attendance record from Newcastle, New Brunswick is but one example of such measures taken throughout the country. (Courtesy Douglas Murray)

When the children recovered, Helen's mother went out to nurse other sick people, sitting up with them and making poultices for their chests. Eventually she got 'flu herself, as did her husband; he was left with a weak heart and was unable to work for several years. The doctor, who lived across the brook from the Murphy family, had the only telephone in the community. In winter he got around to see his patients by horse and pung. Pungs, used in New Brunswick, were elegant sleighs, some of them closed in against the winter winds and painted and decorated with gold scrolls. Buffalo robes kept the passengers cozy and warm.

For the Swim family of Doaktown, on the Miramachi River, the 'flu epidemic had tragic results. Of their three sons, two died — Lloyd, twenty-three, a fourth-year medical student at McGill University, on October 23, and three weeks later, twenty-eight-year-old Earle — both in the space of less than a month.

During the last ten days of September there were a few cases of 'flu at Moncton, but in October it struck in full force with more than three thousand people falling ill. The First Baptist Church opened its Sunday School classrooms to accommodate patients. There were eighty-five deaths, nearly all people under thirty-five years. At Edmunston there were two thousand cases and twenty-three deaths.

Attendance at Sackville's Mount Allison University was down because of the war. During the epidemic classes were continued, although students kept pretty much to the residences to avoid contact with outsiders. At Bartibogue, where they cut spool wood, the death rate was heavy. One man who brought bodies out on a portage sled before the roads froze over was faced with a dreadful task; the water had splashed into the sleigh and the bodies had frozen together. There was no alternative but to chop them apart.

Throughout the province, it was estimated that there had been 35,581 cases and 1,394 deaths.

CENTRAL CANADA

Quebec's first major civilian outbreak was on September 8, 1918, at Victoriaville College. Out of 410 students, 400 got the disease, as did 12 teachers. Although influenza was not a reportable disease, the college observed the kind of care they would have for any contagious disease. With almost all the teachers ill, however, there was little choice but to send home all but the 45 students the school doctor had pronounced too ill to travel. So, more than 350 young people who had either had the disease or had been exposed to it, fanned out across the province. On September 19, a doctor in Levis was called to see one of these boys at his home. After consulting with other doctors, he concluded that the disease was ordinary grippe of medium intensity but that the boy should be kept in quarantine at Quebec City's Civic Hospital.

By September 23, twenty cases of pneumonia had developed at Victoriaville College and there had been six deaths. The same day, nine American sailors died on their ships in port at Quebec City. Forty cases were reported from Trois Rivières, and on the twenty-sixth of the month, the first case appeared in Montreal.

Four hundred soldiers in the camp of engineers at St-Jean were stricken, the total rising to 530 by September 30. A military spokesman said that while the situation remained serious, it was believed the epidemic was now under control and the worst period over. "Only a matter of days now."

By early October, the whole province was affected. One undertaker in Sherbrooke conducted fifteen funerals on one day, and with not enough workers left to run the factories, the town was virtually closed down.

Clearly, the situation was not under control.

The provincial government conferred upon the director of health extraordinary powers, giving him absolute jurisdiction in all the cities, towns, and villages, with action to be taken through local councils of health. In order to avoid unhealthy crowding in public places and on public transport, schools were shut down, and businesses were required to close early. In Montreal, a group of merchants met before the local health council to protest against having to close their establishments at 4:30 P.M. They alleged that their customers all lived locally and therefore did not cause congestion on the streetcars; as well, they asserted, the greatest part of their business was done in the evening. The verdict of the council: to continue closing at 4:30, but to open again at seven in the evening.

At 8:15 on the morning of October 21, 1918, the first passenger train started for Ottawa and Toronto through Montreal's new Tunnel Terminal. Normally it would have been a momentous occasion, but because of the ban on public gatherings no ceremony marked the event.

Influenza was made a reportable disease and, with considerable reluctance because they understood the need of the people to pray, the provincial health board closed churches wherever the epidemic had appeared. Nuns and priests were given permission to work at emergency hospitals.

On October 12, the headline in *Le Devoir* read simply: "Toujours la grippe!" The wrapping of foodstuffs in newspaper or pages of books was officially forbidden, and the public was reminded that doctors were obliged to give death certificates free to the poor.

Dr. Preston McIntyre of Montague, Prince Edward Island was beginning his third year of medical studies at McGill University. When the college closed he got 'flu himself, but it was a mild case and after three days he was able to care for six of his fellow students. Any time they looked out the windows of their residence on Sherbrooke Street they could see trucks passing, carrying rough board coffins; there weren't enough hearses, or enough caskets.

From the dining room of the Strachan home on Prince Arthur Street, the view was of Pine Avenue. During the epidemic there was a constant line of funerals passing along toward Mount Royal Cemetery, so the family drew the drapes at mealtimes. The schools were closed, and young Hilda Strachan Coleman was at home. Wanting her to have fresh air, but fearing infection, her mother sent her out for walks but warned her never to go down to Ste-Catherine Street where there were crowds. To keep their students up to date, teachers at the Trafalgar School for Girls telephoned lessons to their home-bound students. Eileen Peters, who lived on Mountain Street, was sent to play in the back garden to avoid the sight of funerals from Wray's Funeral Parlor on the street below.

On October 21, an all-time high of 201 deaths was reported in Montreal, and on the following day 1,058 new cases had broken out. Priests gave the last rites on the streets during that month of October and paraded the streets with the Sacred Host to bring the

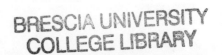

Mass to the people. Led by heralds blowing bugles or ringing bells, they went to doorways, where the faithful knelt to receive the blessing.

Norah Hodgson MacDowell was in the habit of riding every morning before breakfast. On weekends, when she had more time, one of her favorite routes was through Mount Royal Cemetery and over the little mountain where there were a lot of bridle paths. One Saturday morning during October, having ridden into the middle of the cemetery, she found she couldn't get out; there was a funeral on every road leading to a gate.

For burials at the Hawthorn-dale Protestant cemetery, eleven miles from the centre of Montreal, funeral processions ended at the military cemetery on Papineau Avenue near Lafontaine Street. From there coffins were transported by a special funeral car, painted black and discreetly lettered in gold, to Bout de l'Ile. Mourners travelled by regular street-railway car. During the epidemic, the special car carried as many as nine or ten coffins on each trip.

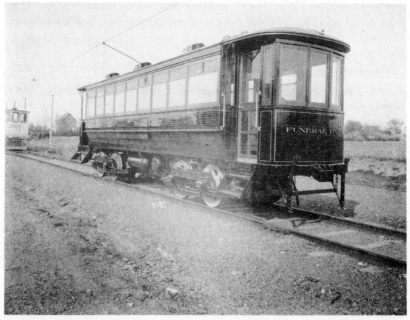

During the epidemic, this special funeral car transported as many as nine or ten coffins a trip to Bout de l'Ile. (Photo courtesy CRHA Archives, MTC Collection)

The Reverend Frederick Lewis Whitley, Priest-in-Charge of the Church of St. James the Apostle, acted as Anglican chaplain at the Guards Emergency Hospital in the Armory of the Canadian Grenadier Guards on Esplanade Avenue opposite Fletcher's Field. Among the patients there was a battalion of young American soldiers en route to England. They were young, homesick, frightened, and very ill; many sad letters had to be written to parents.

A member of the Voluntary Aid Detachment (VAD) of the St. John Ambulance Brigade, Dorothy Macphail Lindsay, also worked at the Grenadier Guards Emergency Hospital. Every morning when she reported for duty she found that several patients had died during the night and new ones had taken their places. There were frequent staff changes too, as one after another came down with 'flu. "Still," she remembers, "I was never aware of any panic. Somehow people stayed steady."

The Department of Marine and Fisheries, which had its own hospital accommodation at most major ports, had none at Montreal. With the threat to shipping posed by the epidemic, at a time when so much depended on getting food and war materials to the troops overseas, officials had to find room quickly for the sixty-some cases of influenza aboard their ships in Montreal harbor on October 22. There had been word from the provincial health board that unless these sick sailors were removed at once from the ships, the ships themselves would be placed under quarantine. There was no room in any of the city hospitals.

Quickly, they made arrangements to take over the Catholic Sailors' Club as a temporary hospital, installing one hundred double-decked bunks on the three floors of the club and staffing it with a medical superintendent, two visiting doctors, two other doctors from the fifth year of medical training at McGill University, two volunteer helpers, graduate nurses night and day, and VADs around the clock. By November 3 and 4, only one seaman had been admitted on each day and by the fourteenth it was decided that as soon as the current patients had been discharged, the emergency facility could be closed. The crisis was, to all intents and purposes, over for the seamen, and shipping had suffered very little disruption.

Around the province, the 'flu became a way of life. At the Algonquin Indian Reserve at Maniwaki, October was a month marked by gloom in every way. The skies lowered, the sun disappeared, and the 'flu came. Marguerite Brascoupe Budge, then nineteen, was the youngest in her family and the last one left at home. She was sick, and her parents were sick. "It was so sad and lonesome, in the mist, with never any sun. We could hear people crying, and children coughing, and the funeral processions passed by with the people wearing black veils over their faces." The incessant tolling of church bells in the town had to be stilled because their sound so upset the patients in hospital.

In Nicolet County three husky young men, all weighing over two hundred pounds, worked as masons under the direction of their father, a man of retirement age. He survived the epidemic, while all three of his sons succumbed.

Along the Dartmouth River, the death rate was high. The men who worked in the lumber mills were among the first to catch the infection; one man, feeling quite recovered, went to the village to do his shopping, came home and ate a hearty meal, and was dead before midnight. But with all the trouble, there was still beauty. Hazel Miller Clark, who lived at Gaspé, went one clear September day to the south shore of the bay with her father to watch the three-masted Norwegian barques come in under full sail. They tacked across the bay to the mills on the north shore. "The sails, the blue skies and the colors on the hills that autumn day in 1918 is a picture I will never forget." The area suffered still another attack of influenza in late February and March of 1920, when many pregnant women died. "It seemed like a witch's curse," Hazel Clark says. "If you gave up, you died."

Another Quebec woman who remembers the atmosphere is Bessie Ticehurst Gahagan, who lived at Ticehurst Corners near the Vermont border. Her memory of the atmosphere that year is not so pleasant: "The sky and air seemed always very yellow."

A young soldier from the parish of Rivière Blanche in Matane County kept a sensitive and moving account of his own illness overseas and his concern for his family at home in Quebec. Arthur Lapointe, his heart heavy with sadness at leaving his beloved family, sailed with the 189th Battalion from Halifax in September 1916, bound for training in England before going to the trenches.

In the front lines at Agny, France on June 30, 1918, the weather was almost unbearably hot and some of the men, a sergeant major, a signaller, and a runner, were sick. Their heads ached and their fevers rose. The signaller rolled on the ground, moaning. One of the soldiers prepared a meal but Lapointe, who a moment earlier had been sharply hungry, could not face the thought of food. The company was due for relief, and when Lapointe had rolled up his pack he climbed out of the dugout. "As I reach the top, my head swims with sudden nausea, everything around me whirls, I totter, then fainting, fall headlong to the ground." His head ached violently when he recovered consciousness. A soldier bathed his forehead with a handkerchief soaked in cold water and, although it helped, he could not find the strength to rise to his feet. Soon more of the men were sick and with only one stretcher bearer, there was no choice but to walk to the aid post, nearly a mile away. "For more than an hour, limp as rags, we drag ourselves through a communication trench, under the broiling afternoon sun. One man can no longer stand erect and crawls on hands and knees. We leave him behind, with a comrade looking after him, until help can be secured."

Later, in Britain for leave and officers' training at Bramshott, the armistice had been signed and Lapointe was ill again — the effect, the battalion medical officer said, of gas inhaled in France. His concern was for his family back in Canada. A letter from home told him that one of his brothers was dangerously ill and would probably not recover; knowing that 'flu was very bad in Quebec, he fretted for lack of news. Five days later a message came, but not by mail. In a dreadful dream his youngest sister, Martine, appeared to him in deep mourning. "She led me to a row of graves and named my brothers and sisters as those the graves enclosed. 'I, too, am dead,' she told me, 'but God in his mercy has allowed me to spend this day with you.' Then the dream faded and I awoke," he chronicled in his diary. Through a letter to a friend from someone in his home town, he learned that one of his sisters and two brothers had indeed died.

When Lapointe at last arrived home in Quebec he was met by his brother and his father; his father's mustache was whiter than he remembered, and there were deep lines in his face that had not been there before. The news was even worse than Lapointe had known; two of his sisters and three of his brothers had been carried off by influenza in the space of nine days. "Dear God, if it was only for this that I came home, why did I not fall in action out there?" he asked, despairing.

Struggling to cope with the ravages of the disease in their province, representatives of the Superior Board of Health requested that Ottawa suspend the application of the unpopular conscription law passed by the Borden government in the spring of 1918. Their representation made the point that transport of conscripts caused dissemination of the 'flu germ, endangering both the conscripts themselves and the people in the areas where they were taken. On October 24 they received word that there would be no further call for conscripts.

In the province of Quebec, as in other areas, figures on the extent of the disease and the number of deaths are uncertain. The best available figures indicate that in Quebec 535,700 people had influenza and 13,880 died. Of those deaths, more than 3,000 were in the city of Montreal.

By the end of the coldest, wettest September Toronto had seen in ninety-seven years, 'flu was firmly established there and all across Ontario. Cities took on a strange, silent air; there were few lights, and masked figures hurried along deserted streets. Dr. Arthur E. Parks was only seven years old, but he remembers the time vividly. "It was as if a black, sombre cloud fell over all. People closed their doors and stayed within to keep their lives. When we did go out we saw black crepe sashes on front doors, and when we heard the church bells ring at St. Alban's we knew another one had died."

The disease was considered to have officially arrived in the city on October 3, 1918. Fifty soldiers were quarantined in the military ward of the General Hospital and visitors were prohibited; by the eighth, half the nursing staff of the Grace Hospital was ill. Western and St. Michael's hospitals had no more room, and two hotels, the Arlington and the Mossop, were revamped as temporary hospitals by a staff largely recruited from city hall workers. They removed carpets, sterilized beds, disinfected mattresses. A request from Washington for three hundred nurses to help out with the 'flu epidemic there had to be refused. Dance halls and schools were closed on the sixteenth. Stores advertised mourning clothes: "A charming veil for a small or medium hat shows small chenille dot on a fine mesh, with border of inch-wide ribbon; 36" long by 16" wide, $1.75." Hosiery, it was pointed out, must match the boots, and mahogany brown was a favored shade. In silk, the price for stockings was a dollar fifty to two dollars; in lisle, fifty cents.

The Dominion of Canada Guarantee & Accident Insurance Company advertised a special sickness policy to cover Spanish Influenza. A nurse in a large department store, with the help of one of the store managers, looked after a whole family all sick at the same time. Newspapers printed hints on keeping well: avoid

Insure Against
Spanish Influenza

Our Special Sickness Policy covers Spanish Influenza.

Pays a weekly indemnity and makes provision for hospital expenses.

It is the most liberal policy you can buy.

For rates apply to any agent of this Company

The Dominion of Canada
Guarantee & Accident Insurance Co.

Canada's Oldest and Strongest Casualty Company.

TRADERS BANK BUILDING, TORONTO.
Phone Main 5388.

Insurance companies advertised special sickness policies to cover Spanish Influenza. (Toronto Daily Star, October 26, 1918. Photo courtesy Metropolitan Toronto Library Board)

getting chilled, keep the hands clean, sleep and work in clean, fresh air, avoid alcoholic stimulants, don't worry — and do not kiss anyone. A similar list of directions from the surgeon general of the United States army suggested: "Avoid tight clothes, tight shoes, tight gloves; seek to make nature your ally, not your prisoner."

PROVINCIAL SECRETARY'S DEPARTMENT

ONTARIO
PROVINCIAL BOARD OF HEALTH

INFLUENZA

PRECAUTIONS

Warning to Health Authorities

"'Health authorities have the power under Section 56, ss. 2, of the Public Health Act to close schools, churches, theatres and other places of assemblage if it is deemed advisable to do so.' Asked what the Board advises regarding this measure, we have said: 'The weight of public health authority is against closing such places, except perhaps in country districts, for the following reasons, viz.: In cities and towns it is impossible to prevent children commingling in the streets and playgrounds where they are without the supervision found in the schools. Hence closing schools is more effective in country districts. Closing schools is economically wasteful, and usually has no influence on the course of an outbreak of disease like influenza. Children are less likely to infect one another in the class-room than in the home or on the playground.'

" As a rule better results will be achieved by a daily inspection of school children, such as for example is maintained in cities like Toronto.

" There is no great danger of spreading the disease in churches, theatres and other assemblages, if these places are well ventilated. In any case, the good derived from closing places of assemblage is more than counterbalanced by the conditions in crowded street cars, railway cars, in large shops and in restaurants where food and dishes may be handled by persons having the disease. It would be just as rational and much more effective to stop all travel on street cars and trains and to stop people from entering shops, eating places, etc., as to close schools, churches, theatres, etc.

" Health officers should do nothing consistent with the welfare of the public, likely to dislocate business or the ordinary affairs of life. They should not be moved from their duty by public clamor, to adopt fussy and ill-advised measures, which only serve to irritate the public and accomplish no useful purpose. If, however, the health officer of any municipality deems it his duty to utilize the section of the Act referred to the Provincial Board will not interfere with him, but the Board does not, for the reasons given, propose to ask its enforcement."

Ontario is confronted by an epidemic of influenza which will in all probability affect more than half of our population. There is a shortage of physicians, nurses, and hospital accommodation. The health and efficiency of the civilian population must be maintained. It is the patriotic duty of every citizen to avoid influenza and keep in good health. To avoid influenza:

Avoid contact with other people so far as possible. Especially avoid crowds indoors, in street cars, theatres, motion-picture houses, and other places of public assemblage.

Avoid persons suffering from " colds." sore throats and coughs.

Avoid chilling of the body or living in rooms of temperature below 65 deg. or above 72 deg. F.

Sleep and work in clean, fresh air.

Keep your hands clean, and keep them out of your mouth.

Avoid expectorating in public places, and see that others do likewise.

Avoid visiting the sick.

Eat plain, nourishing food and avoid alcoholic stimulants.

Cover your nose with your handkerchief when you sneeze, your mouth when you cough. Change handkerchiefs frequently. Promptly disinfect soiled handkerchiefs by boiling or washing with soap and water.

Don't worry, keep your feet warm. Wet feet demand prompt attention. Wet clothes are dangerous and must be removed as soon as possible.

What to do for Influenza and Colds

Oftentimes it is impossible to tell a cold from mild influenza. Therefore:

If you get a cold go to bed in a well ventilated room. Keep warm.

Keep away from other people. Do not kiss anyone. Use individual basins, and knives, forks, spoons, towels, handkerchiefs, soap, wash plates and cups.

Every case of influenza should go to bed at once under the care of a physician. The patient should stay in bed at least three days after fever has disappeared and until convalescence is well established.

The patient must not cough or sneeze except when a mask or handkerchief is held before the face.

He should be in a warm, well ventilated room.

There is no specific for the disease. Symptoms should be met as they arise.

The great danger is from pneumonia. Avoid it by staying in bed while actually ill and until convalescence is fully established.

The after effects of influenza are worse than the disease. Take care of yourself.

This circular advised health authorities against implementing a section of the Public Health Act which empowered them to close places of assemblage. (Photo courtesy Ontario Archives)

The provincial board of health, under no illusions that the province could avoid the epidemic, sent circulars to doctors describing the disease, advising on treatment, and recommending precautions. The board's chief officer took the view that by the time inspection and placarding could be done, a great many people would have recovered and would be kept indoors unnecessarily. Local boards made their own decisions on the closing of churches and schools; generally across the province, public gatherings were discouraged.

By October 9 there were believed to be more than one thousand cases of 'flu in the city, and Dr. C.J. Hastings, medical officer of

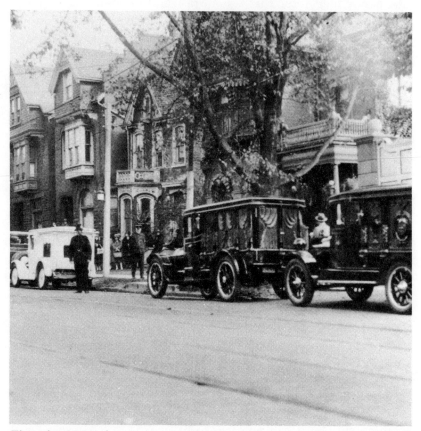

The sight of funeral processions became increasingly common during the epidemic. Shown above are three hearses in front of the Stone Funeral Home in Toronto. White hearses, such as the one in the picture, were for children. (Photo courtesy Donald B. Steenson)

health, ordered the postponement of large gatherings including the Baptist Convention, a meeting of the National Association of Electrical Contractors and Dealers, and a conference of local church workers. He advised the public not to tamper with a healthy body and, leaving all nostrums and gargles alone, to depend upon the advice of their doctors.

In a period of eighteen days, the city suffered 502 deaths. Passengers arriving by train were checked by health officials. Football games were banned./Every available streetcar was put into service to avoid crowding/— a problem since fires in 1912 and 1916 had destroyed 282 cars, and they had not been replaced.

A newspaper noted that a sombre feature of Sunday, October 20, ". . . was the sight of funerals, which are never seen in Toronto on Sunday. These were the casualties in the night, and reminded the thoughtful passer-by that war is not the only destroyer."

On front doors in Toronto, a white sash denoted the death of a child, a gray one a person of middle years, and purple was for a senior citizen. White hearses for children were a common sight in Toronto, remembers John B. Withrow, who had just started to attend John Fisher School on Erskine Avenue. Although Canada's first motorized hearse went into service in Toronto in 1914, there were still horse-drawn hearses everywhere in 1918; wagons and other emergency vehicles were also pressed into service during the epidemic.

Pay for teachers was continued by the board of education, with the caution that they not be paid twice; some had asked for nursing remuneration on top of their teaching salaries. A disproportionate number of married women were ill, as they were unable to take to their beds at the first sign of illness. The *Globe* was frequently late because so many delivery boys were sick.

One Toronto man died at the Base Hospital the same day as his brother died at Camp Mohawk; both had been members of the Royal Air Force. A family on De Grassi Street buried one son and heard that their other son had died in England on the same day, of the same disease.

On October 14, for the first time in three years, the Arraignment Court had no cases to be heard.

During the first two weeks of October, it was estimated that deaths in the city were averaging seventeen a day, but no-one could be sure of the true number because doctors and undertakers were too busy to send in returns. On the twenty-third of the month, 54 out of the health department's staff of 319 were off work. Twenty-two of them were nurses, and 4 were doctors. With people waiting anxiously for the return of men from overseas, newspapers printed notices such as this one, which appeared on October 29: "A troop train carrying 187 men and four officers who reached Canada from overseas on Sunday will arrive in Toronto Tuesday evening or Wednesday morning, if their journey from the Maritime provinces is uninterrupted. For more information, call College 56 and 57."

By October 31, the 'flu had disappeared from the front-page summary of news in the *Globe*, and it was announced that public schools would reopen the following Monday.

In some areas of the province, health authorities considered the public mood and elected to close churches, schools, and theatres at midnight on Thanksgiving Monday so as not to prevent church services or cut off the holiday theatre business. As well, St. Catharines exempted gatherings for the Victory Loan campaign. The annual meeting of the London Curling Club was cancelled.

Undertakers everywhere were desperately busy. The eight cabinet makers in Hamilton worked almost around the clock and every day sent out shipments of caskets to Port Dover, at a transport cost of one dollar each. In London, undertakers took one casket to the cemetery and hurried back to the church to pick up the next. After one funeral at St. Michael's Church, which stood on a high hill, there was no hearse waiting when the people came out; a young girl among the mourners, known to be a bit of a tomboy, put her fingers between her teeth and whistled as though for a taxi. A hearse driver a few streets away heard the signal and hurried to the church.

Eastern Ontario was hard hit. Twelve nurses were sent from Toronto to Renfrew where, on October 5, there were five hundred to six hundred cases and there had been nine deaths. Every factory in town was short of staff, and the large office complement at O'Brien's Limited was down to two workers. At Almonte there were one hundred patients, and eighteen nurses in Ottawa were ill in hospital. The Ottawa board of health urgently requested that all funerals be private. With 350 cases in four days, and 25 deaths, they were in desperate need of more nurses. Theatres, churches, poolrooms, billiard parlors, and bowling alleys were closed. The board of health requested that people walk to work, and those who took the streetcars found the windows wide open whatever the temperature. Stores were open only from 10:00 A.M. to 4:00 P.M., and civil servants were let off at three o'clock for last-minute shopping. The International Plowing Match and tractor demonstration, expected to attract twenty thousand visitors, was cancelled.

Mayor Harold Fisher forwarded to the office of the prime minister a copy of a letter received from a civil servant, complaining that no disinfectant was being used in the offices, the windows were kept closed, and people returned to work whenever they felt like it without a doctor's certificate being required. The writer had been doing volunteer nursing at night and was not afraid to do it, but was afraid of conditions in the office. More than one hundred government clerks were away from work and whole families were sick, with no-one to attend them.

Kingston theatre owners received notices from the medical officer of health that, after consultation with the Kingston Medical Society and under the provisions of the Ontario Health Act, it had been decided that the theatres must close on October 16. The president of the Canadian Theatre Managers' Association responded with an impassioned plea for reconsideration, pointing out the serious hardship such a closing would create for actors, who were not, in general, known to save their money. The medical officer of health remained unmoved, and ten days later notified poolroom proprietors that their establishments too must be closed to the public until further notice.

Travelling players were in difficulty everywhere. Members of the companies of "Furs and Frills," "It Pays to Advertise," and Ben Welch and his Burlesquers waited out the ban in Toronto. Chorus girls from the Stuart-Whyte Company, which had been presenting "Cinderella," didn't waste their time. Some became salesladies, some stenographers, and some got jobs with the hard-pressed telephone company.

The farmers of Lochalsh, near Ripley, were big, strong men of Scottish descent, stubbornly unwilling to accept the idea that they might become ill. A young doctor who had been serving overseas and returned to this, his home community, despaired of getting them to stop work and go home to bed when they had fevers. Dr.

H.O. Howitt had the same problem at Guelph, chiefly with Italians and Austrians, who were splendidly strong and refused to stop work when they became ill. He told the annual meeting of the Canadian Public Health Association in Toronto: "We lost fathers of young families, fathers who felt they had to work on, and young mothers who would not take care of themselves because they thought they had to work or nurse 'for their children's sake.' "

The Ontario School of Agriculture closed its doors. The Polish Camp at Niagara was quarantined. "Not a soldier was seen on the streets last night, except the military police, and the Canadian Camp YMCA was absolutely deserted and in darkness," reported the *Globe*.

/Church closings were not accepted with good grace by everyone. The Reverend Father Trasiuk of Hamilton's St. Stanislaus Church defied the ban and was fined twenty-five dollars. He appealed the case, declaring that the board of health had no right to close churches and citing that the Quebec Act and the Treaty of Paris gave churches freedom of worship without interference from authority. Anglican and Baptist clergymen agreed, but the minister of health stuck to his ruling. Methodist, Presbyterian, and Congregational ministers took the view that the ruling was in the interests of public health, and in the end all submitted./

An Otterville farmer was so desperate for medical attention for his family that he offered to turn over the deed to his homestead to any practitioner who would come, and an Indian woman whose husband had died and who was sick herself paddled her two children by canoe thirty-three miles down the Kapuskasing River — with a six-mile portage — to seek medical help.

October 13 was one of the quietest Sundays ever at Kitchener; the familiar ringing of the church bells was greatly missed. Galt had closed its library, the YMCA, ice-cream parlors, shoe-shine parlors, candy stores, furniture stores, second-hand stores, and Chinese cafes. People observed the bans on public gatherings, but they still had to go out to buy food. Even that became a problem. At one stage every food store on the east side of Galt, except for the Red and White Gray's General Store at the corner of Lincoln and McNaughton, was closed because the proprietors were ill.

The Indian village of Sand Point, on Lake Nipigon, had fifty-eight people ill and five deaths — out of a population of seventy. At Fort William and Port Arthur, now Thunder Bay, the first cases appeared on October 7, when two employees of the Canada Car Company returned from Montreal sick. Ten days later public meetings were banned. As the epidemic grew, scarlet fever broke out as well. At Erin, there was diptheria as well as influenza.

Influenza spread through the Sault Ste. Marie district after a visit of a man from Ottawa. He stayed at a lumber camp at Searchmont for a couple of days and after his departure, sixteen cases were reported in the camp. The body of one of the men who died was ordered buried immediately instead of being shipped to his home in Montreal. All members of the Harry family of Sault Ste. Marie, mother, father, and four children, were ill. Mrs. Susan Harry had serious bedsores and was placed on a rubber mattress filled with water, a new treatment at the time. Her recovery in hospital took two years; to pay for the drugs she required, her husband had to mortgage their home. She eventually had four more children, and lived to the age of seventy-eight years.

Nurse Anna McCrea, who looked after the Harry family, was a revered figure in the Sault Ste. Marie area for her work with newcomers from Italy. "She taught literally hundreds to speak English and to adjust to life in the New World. Later she was honored by having a school named after her," says Kathleen Harry Russell.

One man cared for by Anna McCrea weighed 250 pounds. Delirious from his high fever, as many people were, he jumped out of an upstairs window and ran away into the snow. He did not survive.

When the epidemic finally passed through Ontario, rough statistics placed the number of cases at about 300,000; the number of deaths was recorded as 8,705.

THE PRAIRIE PROVINCES

On September 30, 1918, a group of sick soldiers was removed from a troop train in Winnipeg. They were placed in isolation at a convalescent home belonging to the IODE (the Imperial Order

Daughters of the Empire), where, on October 3, two of them died. On the same day, Winnipeg's first civilian death took place.

It was decided to take precautionary measures. The University of Manitoba and all the colleges in Winnipeg and St-Boniface were closed. On October 12, Dr. A.J. Douglas, Winnipeg's medical health officer, placed a ban on public meetings and suggested that health officers of the various districts throughout the province do the same. "In view of what has happened in cities to the east and south, we must not put up our hands and say 'It is an act of God!' " he warned. The wearing of masks, while not required by law, was advised, and a fifty-dollar fine or a jail term was instituted for anyone spitting on the street.

Newspapers supported the measures taken by the health authorities and so, generally, did the churches, although pamphlets were circulated condemning their closure as showing a lack of faith in God. A Baptist minister refuted the assertion, saying: "To pray for immunity from the plague while ignoring natural precautions is impiety itself."

An attempt by the Women's Civic League to have bakers' bread wrapped was unsuccessful; it was decided that unwrapped bread would not spread disease and that the extra expense involved in wrapping would be unjustified. Reports of a rise in juvenile delinquency suggested that children, idle because schools were closed, had too much time to get into mischief. The restriction of gatherings of more than six or eight people cut down severely on all celebrations, including weddings. Not everyone obeyed the ban; one mother complained that her children had been invited to Hallowe'en parties and were very annoyed when she would not allow them to attend.

The family of a Winnipeg man returning from overseas ignored the instruction to stay home from the railway station. Not allowed to approach the disembarking passengers, they waved to him from a distance and went dejectedly home to await his discharge from the army receiving centre. He escaped the 'flu, but his wife caught it.

Residential institutions and orphanages were hard hit by 'flu, with 107 out of 151 students ill at the School for the Deaf, and more than 100 cases and 5 deaths at the Home for the Friendless.

Moving picture house operators, in October showing "The White Man's Law," "Vive La France," and "M'Liss" with Mary Pickford, among others, found themselves in financial trouble when they had to close but were still obliged to pay rent to their landlords. "The local theatres do not wish to take the matter up with Ottawa, feeling assured that the owners of the buildings fully appreciate the serious position in which they have been placed through no fault of their own. . . ." reported the *Manitoba Free Press* for October 17. They continued to disinfect their theatres daily, in hopes of an early reopening. Their protests were evidently effective, to some degree at least, because in January 1919 the provincial government voted to allow them to hold back 25 percent of taxes on ticket sales throughout the following six months, the money to be used to compensate the three or four hundred employees affected.

By October 13, the death toll in the city was 8 and there were 72 new cases, bringing the total up to 330. The speedy onset of this treacherous malady was brought home to Winnipegers when a man who lived on Flora Street died just three hours after he had noticed the first symptoms. By the end of the month there were 1,462 cases and 50 deaths, and the newspapers reported that the epidemic was beyond control; yet early in November the *Winnipeg Tribune* felt able to headline: "Skiddoo, Flu! We're about rid of you!" and by the end of the month, the ban on public gatherings in the city had been lifted.

"Winnipeg — in the healthy and sheltered middle of Canada; several thousand solid miles and many well protected water miles from the nearest fighting ground of the late great war; out of range of the submarines or the exploding munition ships; never in its history visited by great earthquake or cyclone . . ." exulted the *Winnipeg Free Press.*

But, though the ban on public gatherings had been lifted and the city had begun to sigh with relief, the 'flu had not yet given up entirely. After the schools had reopened, a celebration was held at the Oblate Fathers' Juniorate in St-Boniface to honor a father who had reached his centenary. A play was staged, and during the performance a student became suddenly ill. Leon Jalbert, playing a sinister role, made his entrance slowly, onto a dimly lit stage, brandishing a dagger over his head. As he spoke his dramatic lines he felt his face flush, but assumed it was just stage fright.

The director, however, noted the suspiciously red face and, when it was found that the boy did indeed have a fever, he was sent to hospital to recover from 'flu — in a cold, horse-drawn paddy wagon, the only ambulance available.

An estimate of cases in Winnipeg by the end of January put the figure at 12,863, with 824 deaths.

Chautauqua, the travelling entertainers whose clusters of brown tents were a familiar sight across Canada from 1917 to 1935, had to stop their shows when the ban was placed on public assembly. The players who lived near enough went home, while others stayed on wherever they happened to be. Some lent a hand with emergency nursing, while others waited out the time in hotels. Chautauqua's management eventually had to admit defeat, and performances were cancelled for the year.

Cora Hamilton Lenton, who lived with her parents on a farm five miles north of Miami, remembers that the disease struck so rapidly there that people didn't dare go into other houses or even into town except when absolutely necessary. Her family used to phone in their grocery order and wait in the car for the boxes to be brought out. Two members of the household were very ill and they were fortunate in being able to get a trained nurse. Two young mothers in the immediate family died, one of them leaving a five-day-old baby and the other a two-year-old daughter. The Hamilton family took the little girl into their home, where she remained until she married. "People can hardly realize what we went through then," says Cora Hamilton Lenton.

In The Pas, the undertaker became ill with 'flu himself and had to call on a friend to take over the work. Jean Mastái Poirier was a contractor, not an undertaker, but he had had some training in his youth when he had been preparing to enter the priesthood. He built caskets in the kitchen of his home and, according to the custom of the time, covered the ones for white victims with cloth and painted those for Indians with black paint. He kept his nine-year-old daughter Florence busy making little satin pillows for the caskets. The pressure under which he worked became so intense that often the parish priest would bring him, ahead of time, measurements of someone not expected to live. Those who died in isolated country areas could not always be buried immediately so their bodies were placed on the roofs of log cabins, out of reach of animals, to be buried in the spring.

There were two doctors at The Pas. One travelled by horse and cutter, and the other by dogteam or on the muskeg train of the Hudson's Bay Railway to surrounding small settlements. St. Anthony's Hospital, run by the Grey Nuns, Sisters of Charity, was soon overcrowded and the Avenue Hotel was taken over for emergency accommodation. Florence Poirier Gudgeon recalls: "It brought out the meaning of being a friend, a neighbor. In The Pas, no-one was neglected or forgotten." Two young men, one of them later to be Florence's husband, drove a canvas-covered sleigh which served as an ambulance. On their rounds they went into homes where people were ill to fill the water barrel, to carry in wood, and to keep the stoves going. They also delivered pots of soup made by the people of the community.

At Swan River, John Lambert got word that his neighbor on the next farm was ill; although he drove immediately to town to fetch him medicine, the man died the next day. George Barker, who later became chief of his people, was working on the boat *Majestic,* which plied Lake Winnipeg, when the 'flu struck that area. With most of the dozen crew sick, they docked near the present Provencher Bridge. Barker heard the church bells ring and watched the black trucks used as hearses passing by. When they took to the water again, only five of the original twelve were left.

A young woman in Brandon, caring for her sick husband in an upstairs apartment, shivered at the eerie sound of a cart rattling by in the street below. It was collecting the bodies of the dead.

Men who had survived the war sometimes came safely home, only to succumb to this new enemy. One of these was Canada's youngest-ever winner of the Victoria Cross, eighteen-year-old Alan McLeod of Stonewall, Manitoba. When his plane was fired upon by eight enemy triplanes, he shot down three of them and, despite multiple wounds, kept on fighting until a bullet penetrated the gas tank and set his plane on fire. He clambered out onto the wing and flew the craft from there until he crashed in No Man's Land. Six months later, back in Canada to a hero's welcome, he contracted influenza and died in his home town.

In Saskatchewan, the first Regina resident to succumb was a drayman who lived on Robinson Street North; he had been sick about a week and died on October 6, 1918 in the General

Hospital. Two days later, by order-in-council, influenza was made a reportable disease across the province, with all cases to be isolated and quarantined.

In Regina it was decided to keep the library open, in the absence of other entertainment to which the public was accustomed. Streetcar service was cut back because so many motormen and conductors were away sick, and Sunday runs were cancelled altogether for the duration of the ban on church services. People were urged to take their cars out on Sundays to enjoy the benefit of the fresh air without fear of being considered unpatriotic during the wartime gasoline shortage.

The city had planned a noisy launching for its October 29 Victory Loan campaign, with steam whistles, fire engines, and automobile horns, but because of the number of sick people, quiet was essential. The organizers of the six-million-dollar appeal settled instead for only the appearance on downtown streets of the Victory Loan Regina Tank. Canvassers going door-to-door for funds were asked to gather data on the epidemic at each home they visited and to report their findings to the Central Health Bureau.

By the end of October, two thousand Regina people had 'flu.

Train service around the province had to be cut because so many railway employees were sick. Daily trains from Regina to Colonsay and to Weyburn were reduced to thrice weekly, as was the Moose Jaw to North Portal service. The number of sleeper cars on the Trans-Canada express was reduced. E.W. Beattie, president of the Canadian Pacific Railway, urged the public to curtail unnecessary train travel.

Mrs. Charles Wilson of Limerick recalled those long-ago days in an article in the *Assiniboia Times* of June 15, 1955: "While the doctor was hors de combat, we did as the pioneers always did, we made do with what we had, and thanked God that we had so much." The whole community turned out to help, and schools and homes were turned into emergency hospitals. When the Chinese proprietor of the town laundry could no longer get staff, volunteers bought a gasoline washer and borrowed a mangle; two young army men did a huge wash every day and in the evening took the clothes and bedding back to the hospital, dried and folded. One man bought a Chevrolet car, put a Red Cross symbol on the window, and patrolled a large area every day; another, whose wife had been buried the day before, reported for duty as usual at the emergency hospital at seven o'clock in the morning.

In the week of October 17, the 'flu spoiled a proud record: the *Oxbow Herald*, which hadn't missed an issue in fifteen years, had to suspend publication because so many of the staffers were sick.

The first cases of 'flu appeared in Saskatoon on October 15, and on the seventeenth, theatres and schools were closed. Emmanuel College and part of Sutherland School were taken over as emergency hospitals; teachers operated a food kitchen at Victoria School. Houses were placarded. In all, about two hundred and fifty Saskatoon people died.

At nearby Rosetown, the morgue was so crowded with bodies that the undertaker had to take over the lumber yard as well.

One travelling salesman who kept trying to conduct his route called at a store at Paradise Hill and found both the proprietor and his wife dead. Nearby, he found three Indians lying dead, and not far away a young man worked alone to dig graves for his parents and his brother and sister. At Witchekan Lake, an entire threshing crew was found dead.

In contrast to the people who were stricken suddenly, H.E. Petersen's illness came along gradually. He was pitching bundles for a threshing outfit southwest of Radville when he began to feel a cold coming on. Next day, when he couldn't face the idea of breakfast, his boss gave him a cup of coffee with a stiff measure of brandy in it. He went out to the fields but couldn't work. It wasn't just a head cold and a backache; it was the 'flu.

Stanley Hurst, whose father was elevator agent for the United Grain Growers at Stenen, was seven that year. As he crossed the Canadian Northern railway tracks between his home and his father's office, he passed the hardware store where he could see piles of coffins in their wooden cases; day by day, the pile diminished and people had to begin building them at home.

The nearest doctors were twenty miles to the east and the same distance south. They were called from Stenen's only telephone, at the King George V Hotel, or they were summoned by telegraph; sometimes a livery stable operator went to get one of them with a team and cutter, and sometimes the section crew brought them into town by speeder car. From their home, the Hurst family could hear the sound of the speeder cutting through the icy Saskatchewan night, and they would wonder with a shudder who was sick this time. Train crews carried prescriptions to Canora and brought the medicine back on the next run.

The dirt roads of the area around Stenen were sometimes deeply rutted, and in wet weather horses and buggies and the cars of the time, Model T Fords, Chevrolet 490s, Gray Dorts, McLaughlins, and Overlands, had to ford the streams. In winter the cars were put away, and residents relied on cutters and sleighs, and on train travel.

At last, a medical officer was hurried out of a group of army personnel on its way home and rushed to Stenen, without even an opportunity to get into civilian clothing. Making his rounds by horse and cutter, driven by the livery stable proprietor, he was a welcome addition indeed to the community — especially when outbreaks of diptheria, scarlet fever, and some smallpox followed the 'flu. He was able, too, to arrange for a druggist to set up business in the town.

Country residents were struck hard. The residents of a Ukrainian settlement nearby, which suffered a lot of deaths, followed a custom of their homeland by burying their dead at night. As they passed through the village toward their cemetery on the north side, they sang dirges that sent chills along the spines of the listeners. Eventually they were persuaded to take another route.

During the first three months of the 'flu epidemic, 3,906 Saskatchewan people died. By the following April, the total had risen to 4,821.

Officials in Regina had been warned by Winnipeg colleagues that there were infected soldiers on a troop train bound from Quebec City to Vancouver, and they passed the word on up the line. Calgary's medical health officer, Dr. C.S. Mahood, was on hand when the train arrived at the station. He removed fifteen men who had sickened during the trip from Regina and took them personally to an isolation ward at Sarcee Military Camp, careful not to let them come in contact with anyone else in the hope that the epidemic would not spread. It was three o'clock in the morning of October 2, 1918; the influenza epidemic had arrived in Alberta, and Mahood's precautions had been in vain. In less than a week not only had the disease spread within the military hospital, but other cases had appeared around the city.

/ Mahood attacked the problem boldly. There was no provision under the Alberta Health Act for quarantine of influenza cases, but he imposed a modified quarantine on October 16 anyway/It was difficult to make it work. Sometimes people were not sure whether they had influenza or just a cold, and sometimes they were reluctant to admit to having what was obviously the 'flu because it meant stopping day-to-day activities for everyone in the house; whoever earned the money could not go out even if he felt well. Therefore, many didn't call for medical attention when they should have.

On October 18 schools, churches, and theatres were closed, and public meetings were banned. From the twenty-fifth of the month citizens were required to wear gauze masks outside their own homes, although many wore them only when they thought a policeman might be looking. To add to Calgary's general misery, eighteen hundred street railway workers went out on strike and halted public transportation.

There was, however, an occasional bright spot. Charlotte Atkins Elliott, who had become accustomed to using the telephone very little because of wartime restrictions, found it nice to be able to call friends in good conscience during a time when get-togethers were forbidden. But even that pleasure didn't last long. Soon the telephone company requested people to refrain from using telephones unnecessarily because the service was needed on an emergency basis and many operators were away sick.

No work was accepted by dry cleaners, although articles already on hand were disinfected and could be picked up. An unused hospital was pressed into service for 'flu patients, as were a number of schools. Soup kitchens were set up, and volunteers took their turn.

The Hudson's Bay Company announced that not only were they keeping their store properly disinfected for the protection of the public, but their staff had been wearing masks three days before the order came out. No amount of publicity, however, could convince people that for maximum effectiveness the masks should be worn no more than two hours and then should be boiled before the next wearing to avoid germs multiplying in the

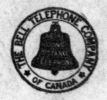

An Urgent Appeal
to All Telephone Users

The Spanish Influenza has caused a very serious shortage in our operating force.

In order to insure prompt and efficient handling of important Government calls and calls to physicians, dealing with the epidemic, the public is requested:

(1) To make only the most urgent and necessary calls.

(2) To refrain, as far as possible, from special appeals to Managers, whose entire time should be given to the supervision of their central offices.

(3) To show consideration of those operators who, despite their increased tasks necessitating overtime work, are loyally giving of their best endeavors.

This is a frank statement of the conditions. We are confident that only a word to the public in such a situation is necessary.

The Bell Telephone Company of Canada

Telephone companies across the country were forced to beg the public's indulgence with advertisements such as this one from The Bell Telephone Company. (The Globe, Toronto, Ontario, 19 October, 1918. Photo courtesy Ontario Archives) warm damp cloth. One Calgarian described how they cared for their masks: "We wore the same one all day at work, then when we got home at night we washed it out and hung it by the fire to be 'sterilized' for wearing next day." If the masks caused more infection than they prevented, as some declared, at least they prevented the custom of spitting on the street. Store-bought masks cost between five and twenty-five cents or, if tailor-made, thirty-five cents. Enterprising Victory Bond salesmen had the legend "Buy a Bond" printed across the gauze.

For more than a month George Cardiff, a driver for the Alberta Box Company, transported only rough oblong boxes in his horse-drawn wagon; Calgary was out of coffins.

As the number of 'flu cases diminished, businessmen who had lost vast amounts of money during the shut-down began to protest that the epidemic was over and it was time to get back to normal. Unwillingly, authorities bowed to the pressure and lifted the bans on November 23, after no new cases had been reported. Dances were resumed, but could last only two hours, and dancers were ordered to remain a yard away from their partners. Dr. Mahood warned that there would probably be a recurrence, and early in December he was proved right; a second wave began, and lasted until almost the end of January.

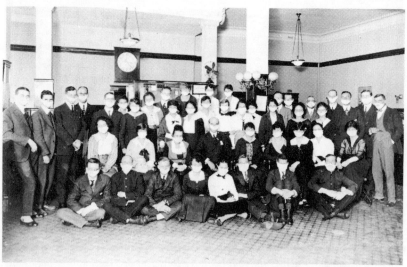

Shown above is the staff of Calgary's Canadian Bank of Commerce wearing anti-influenza masks. (Photo courtesy Glenbow Archives)

Thanks to publicity about the 'flu epidemic in Calgary, the United States army got the services of two Canadians. Ed and Bert Johnson, from southern Alberta, wanted to go to war but did not want to die of 'flu before ever getting to the trenches, so they decided they would be safer to go straight south and join up with the Americans instead of going through Calgary's enlistment centre. They had family ties in the United States and anyway, "It was all the same war, wasn't it?" Neighbors thought they had a good idea and finally a group of ten young men set up a camp near Hailstone Butte, equipping themselves to make a run for the United States.

Five of the group backed out, and three more decided to wait out the war back in the hills. That left just Edwin Johnson, twenty-four, and his brother, twenty-three-year-old Bert, to undertake the ninety-mile ride south through wooded country and across rivers and creeks to the border crossing into Montana. They sold their horses to a ranger, eventually getting them returned when he was jailed by Canadian authorities for smuggling. The ranger wasn't sure he believed the unlikely story these two Canadians told, so he escorted them to Cut Bank, Montana and turned them over to the sheriff there. That night they spent in jail, with the cell door open, and next day, in the sheriff's custody, they rode the further sixty-five miles south to the enlistment centre at Choteau, Montana. There the two surprised Canadians found they were heroes, and recipients of speeches and bouquets from the town stage. "We were the only two volunteers on the last troop train to Fort Lewis, Washington," said Ed Johnson. He became, ironically, a military policeman, and his brother was made a machine gunner. Several months after the war's end, the two Canadian "draft dodgers" received honorable discharges from the army.

Influenza didn't strike Edmonton until October 19, but on that day forty-one cases appeared. The city had been taking all the precautions it could; schools were already closed, and churches and other public gathering places followed. Later in the month, stores were permitted to be open only between 10:00 A.M. and 3:00 P.M., and the board of health set up a central point to organize nurses and volunteer helpers.

The disease hit so fast that a city baker, Tom Caufield, claimed: "You could be talking to a man on the street, turn around and

walk down the street. You'd look back and he had fallen over."
The order to wear masks in public was rescinded after store hours
were shortened, but during its lifetime street railway employees
were empowered to call police to eject anyone failing to wear a
mask. The sight of masks bothered people. One woman said: "It
made me delirious . . . seeing spooks in every corner of the room."
Spitting on the streets was strictly forbidden and the once-familiar
spittoons were outlawed.

Hudson's Bay store employees, all wearing the required masks,
were subjected to "sick parades" three times a day. Parents kept
their children in the house. One Edmonton doctor remembers that
he sat at an upstairs window of his house on 124th Street,
watching pedestrians and wishing he could go out to play.

On October 21, fifty-seven members of the Canadian branch of
the expedition to Siberia, undertaken by Allied countries during
the Bolshevik Revolution, were taken from a train passing through
Edmonton en route to Vancouver and quarantined at the

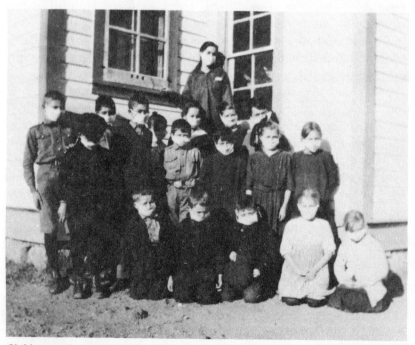

*Children at Fairgrove School, near Sedgewick, Alberta attended school during the
epidemic, but wore cheesecloth masks soaked in hydrogen peroxide as a defense
against germs. (Photo courtesy Frank Snowsell)*

Connaught Armories. One man who was later to be a member of that expedition was John Stewart, who joined the Royal North West Mounted Police in Edmonton during August 1918. He was training at Regina when he developed influenza. When first admitted to hospital he was the only patient on the ward, but by nightfall half a dozen more had joined him. In just a few days he was released, feeling fine, but in less than a week he was back in hospital suffering from pneumonia. Delirious, he lost all track of time. Bodies were removed by a grave-digging detail and at one point a grave was ordered for him — "But I survived." When he was released from hospital, his normal weight of 150 pounds had dropped to 120 pounds.

With Squadron "B," he was sent to Vancouver and then to Vladivostok, Siberia aboard the ship *Monteagle*, which carried both horses and men. During his stint in Siberia, which lasted from December 1918 until July 1919, he attended some of Raymond Massey's shows in Vladivostok while on leave; Massey was serving there with the Canadian Artillery.

After Stewart's discharge to pension in 1952, he wrote to the force headquarters in Ottawa asking for all papers relating to his service. Among the documents was a will he had signed, without knowing it, during the time he was so ill in Regina.

All throughout Alberta, schools were turned into emergency hospitals, and volunteers did their best with what they had to work with. Sometimes they had trained nurses to direct the work, but more often they did not. When schools closed at Granum, Jeanette Huntley Holms, a teacher, went to help the Boyle family. At first three were very ill, then four. Despite the very strict quarantine in effect, the woman living next door rose above the danger to her own family and slipped in after dark to help the young teacher tend her patients. "The people were so good. They even seemed inspired. 'Be your brother's keeper' was practiced more then than I have ever seen since," Jeanette Holms remembers.

Community newspapers printed column after column of 'flu illnesses and deaths, but the Grande Prairie *Herald* made a point of noting, too, the happy news of recoveries. In that town a fifty-dollar fine for not wearing a mask was instituted. Under Local and General News Notes, the paper reported without comment that two of the nurses from the Kathryn Prettie Hospital had gone to Edmonton on the last train, "leaving them rather shy of help during the present trouble."

Medical students were assigned to ride on trains to make sure that passengers wore masks. In more than one hundred prairie towns, travellers were not allowed to de-train unless they agreed to stay where they were until the epidemic was over. Some communities, including Lethbridge, instituted actual quarantines around their boundaries. At Alliance, southeast of Edmonton, townspeople manned stations at the roads leading into town, halting visitors and carrying messages in and replies back. For nearly two months, from November 2 until the end of December, the town operated in isolation from the rest of the world. The doctor, thirty years old and married only three weeks, was the town's first death in the epidemic. Funerals were held outdoors. With no priest nearer than Castor, across the Battle River, the Reverend Mr. Clegg enlisted the help of lay people from the town to conduct suitable services for Catholic people.

The ban was partially lifted at the end of November, just to allow farmers from the district to come and go, but visitors from

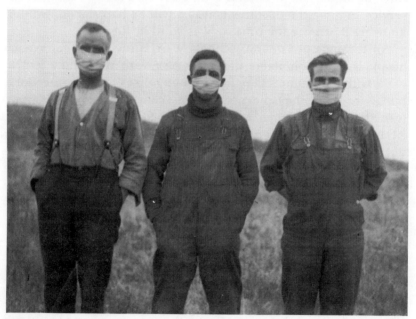

Three prairie farmers wear surgical masks to ward off Spanish Influenza. (Photo courtesy Public Archives Canada, PA 25025)

other centres were still not admitted. Alliance returned to normal at the end of the year, with the school fumigated and ready for classes on January 7, but the respite didn't last. In March and April the epidemic came back, worse than ever. By then the town had a doctor again and, under his direction, the hotel was turned into an emergency hospital. Public gatherings were banned once more, but the quarantine was not reimposed; while patients occupied the upper floors of the hotel, patrons came and went freely through the lobby. It was not until April 26, 1919 that the last patient went home.

When it was all over in Alberta, statisticians estimated that one in ten people in the province who caught the disease died of it, more than thirty-three hundred altogether.

THE PACIFIC COAST

In a normal year the citizens of Corbin, British Columbia could expect at least six feet of snow. But 1918 was not in any respect a normal year. The fall was mild, so mild that even though the ground was frozen, dust blew across the mountains from the prairies and settled on the mountain peaks, glowing a strange, dull red.

Life was good in Corbin. In that heyday of mining, everyone had a job supplying coal to the Spokane International Railway and to the Canadian Pacific Railway, they lived in company houses, and shopped at the company store and the town's one butcher shop. There was plenty to do for recreation. In winter there were parties and dances with an orchestra and a brass band, and in summer, tennis and baseball were played on lots dug out of the sides of the mountain with teams and scrapers, and finished smooth by pick and shovel. Or, they played in or cheered on the soccer teams organized by the many Scottish and English miners. An active league of teams from Corbin, Michel, Coal Creek, and Fernie, in British Columbia, played against Hosmer, Blairmore, Coleman, and Hillcrest across the border in Alberta.

The population of fifteen hundred was made up of many nationalities: Italians, Poles, Slavs, Ukrainians, Russians, and British. Many of the newcomers spoke only a smattering of English, but they soon learned enough to get jobs. One Russian miner who applied at the company offices for his mining papers was asked: "What would you do first thing down the mine?" "Load some coal." "Then what would you do?" "Load some more coal." That was all the official needed to know, and the man got his papers.

Bootlegging was big business in the Crowsnest Pass, despite the several policemen posted there for that very reason and for war-time surveillance of the many foreign-born residents. Imaginative purveyors took liquor back and forth across the Canada-U.S. border in spare tires — successfully, until they got too greedy and began using large truck tires as spares on their Packard cars. The change inspired curiosity at the border. Others transported the precious booty in the body cavities of frozen beef carcasses. Less risky was to make the booze at home. Potatoes were a good source, but left an unpleasant aftertaste, so a more popular base was the pailful or two of grain left in boxcars brought to Corbin to be loaded with coal for Vancouver. It was distilled in big wooden barrels with water, yeast, and sometimes a few raisins or prunes to give it body; when it had dripped through copper pipes into kegs, this brew was 100 percent overproof, strong enough to make a man walk down the street talking to himself. It was to play an important role in the life of at least one Corbin man that fall, a lumberjack called Missouri Bill.

Jack Cumberland, a young Englishman who started work at the mines as a boy of fourteen picking rocks from screens, had by 1918 graduated to the job of carpenter's helper at $2.50 for a nine-hour day. Like everyone else, he had read in the Calgary newspapers reports of the dreaded Spanish Influenza that was sweeping the world and making its way westward in Canada, but in the clean dry air of Corbin, more than five thousand feet above sea level, the danger seemed remote. Then, on a sunny afternoon in early October, a peddler stepped from the Fernie train carrying his sample case of yard goods and ribbons — and the 'flu germ.

Overnight, half the town was sick. One of the first to catch the disease was the doctor; he had just time to prescribe: "Stay in bed, take Epsom salts, and more Epsom salts." Cumberland was called on to help convert the dance hall to an emergency hospital for the bachelor miners. Hastily, the workmen covered rough log walls with building paper for insulation and erected makeshift bunks.

Coal-fired stoves provided heat, and the hospital was in business.

Their first patient was Missouri Bill. Scorning the doctor's advice to take Epsom salts, he persuaded Cumberland to keep him supplied instead with the powerful locally-made moonshine, so strong that when set alight it burned with a blue flame like brandy. For Missouri Bill the cure worked, and after his recovery he spread the word that the only sure way to cope with the 'flu was to hang your hat on the bedpost, go to bed, and drink moonshine until you could see two hats.

Three of the other bachelor patients did not fare so well. Ignoring warnings to stay in bed, as soon as they felt a little better they got up and ate heavy meals. It was a fatal error. Cumberland's help was needed again, this time to dig graves. The ground, filled with fist-sized boulders, was frozen solid. He built a big fire to thaw the frozen earth and dug a hole six feet deep and ten feet across.

Everyone in town who was well enough to get around helped his neighbor. With the doctor sick, the mine engineer made the rounds from house to house, checking temperatures and making sure everyone had what was needed. Although families on both sides of them were sick, no-one in Cumberland's household caught the disease, and they busied themselves carrying coal and wood, and stoking fires, for less fortunate people. Jack Cumberland remembers: "In those days nobody thought twice about taking risks; we just all helped out."

The disease spread rapidly across the province. The provincial board of health issued an immediate order-in-council banning public meetings, a ruling which was not readily accepted in all localities; the board noted later that those areas slow in adopting the measure had suffered a higher death rate. The use of masks was optional.

Cranbrook opened the old Wentworth Hotel as an auxiliary hospital and used the Leask house on Garden Avenue for a nurses' home. The Cranbrook *Herald* was having problems: "Part of the staff is sick, the linotype has the 'flu and the paper is being set by hand," they announced.

Rural schools at Kelowna remained open, but the town schools closed and public gatherings were banned. An isolation hospital was opened in the old school beside the Presbyterian church. The

What a Closed Town Means

STORES, industries and offices "carry on" business as usual.
Every place of assembly closed, every meeting stopped, all public amusement curtailed. Order effective this morning.

This will entail a heavy loss to lessees of halls, to caterers, theatres, dance halls, pool rooms, auctioneers, rinks and many other businesses.

Even the august sessons of the city council are at an end until further notice.

The police court may not close.

Laundry strikers cannot assemble to discuss grievances. Lodges cannot carry on their secret rites.

Unions cannot call members together, but the order will not interfere greatly with the conduct of their affairs.

Victory Loan drive to go right on, with vigorous outdoor programme. The great parade will take place as planned on October 28.

Y. M. C. A. activities postponed; Y. W. C. A. residents hold house parties.

Public library closed, but staff will work on cataloguing.

Curtailment of all amusement outside the home foreshadows revival of the old fashioned parlour game, family song fest, talk fest, and good old hospitality.

Canadian club luncheon to Lieut.-Col. Purney and Lieut.-Col. Hendrie called off, and also Board of Trade luncheon to W. A. Blair.

Numerous auction sales deferred, including seven in one week by one auctioneer.

Interesting legal situation over hall rent for cancelled meetings, and wages of employees in public meeting places.

Many city ministers will publish their sermons in the Sun. Others will make personal calls on members of their congregation; and still others will keep in touch with them by telephone.

102nd Battalion club banquet postponed.

No indoor swimming nor gymnasiums; physical culture will be strictly an individual affair.

University of British Columbia classes dispersed.

Total of 900 Cases of Influenza Reported in City Up to Midnight; Death Roll Is 32.

280 NEW CASES YESTERDAY

Another School Converted Into Hospital; Mayor to See that Closing Order Is Enforced.

TOTAL number of cases, (civilian only), 900.
Deaths, civilian, 19; military, 13.
Cases, civilian, reported yesterday, 280.
Cases, civilian, reported previous day, 90.
Number of military cases, censored.
Order closing city received by Mayor Gale from Hon. J. D. MacLean, provincial secretary, at 5.50 p. m. yesterday, to go into effect this morning.
General business life of city not effected by closing.
Cases continue to be mild as a general rule.
Hospital accommodation is being increased.

WITH a total of 900 reported cases of Spanish influenza among civilians up to last midnight and the likelihood of many more unreported cases, Vancouver today becomes a closed city, thus preventing by forbidding assemblies of people, the spread of the disease, if that is possible. The military authorities refused last night to make public the number of cases among soldiers.

One gratifying feature which continues to be a source of great satisfaction to Dr. Underhill, medical health officer, and the other physicians who are coping with the plague, is that the mortality is exceptionally low, the known deaths among civilians being but 19 and the total number of military deaths 13. The figures as to deaths among civilians stricken with the disease may fall short of the actual total, as the health department is too busily engaged handling the cases of illness to check up on the death reports.

The order closing the city was received by wire from Hon. J. D. MacLean, provincial secretary, at 5.50 p.m. yesterday. It read as follows:

Mayor Gale, Vancouver:
On the recommendation of the secretary of the provincial board of health, the government has decided to make the influenza regulations apply today to Vancouver. Full text of the order will be forwarded.

J. D. MacLEAN.

The following places consequently will be closed today, to remain closed indefinitely:

Churches, or places used for devotional exercise, schools, public or private, or classrooms, public libraries, theatres, moving picture houses, dance halls, poolrooms, gymnasiums, skating rinks and swimming pools public fairs or exhibitions, public auctions, lodge or fraternal society meetings, union meetings, literary or social clubs, and public or private dance halls.

CLOSING ORDER SENDS CITY BACK TO SIMPLE LIFE

WHAT all the simple life preachers failed to do with years of talking, the influenza germ has done in two short weeks. Whether Vancouver likes it or not, it has been converted over-night into an apostle of the simple life.

No more theatres to divert the minds of the city's workers—also non-workers. No more lectures to improve these same minds. No more fiery mass meetings to set the world right in questions of politics, religion, economics and all.

Such being the case it is likely that families will commence the "closed period" by sitting down to get mutually acquainted. The mother who has been given to sighing that she was "too tired to go to that meeting, but wouldn't feel right if she stayed at home" will settle herself with a free mind and perchance a mending basket.

The father who has wandered forth in the damp chill night to seek the fraternal fellowship of the lodge meeting, will now, remembering that there is no such meeting, dislodge his small [...]

HEAVY FINANCIAL LOSS IS CAUSED BY PEREMPTORY ORDER

IT is only when a closing order goes into effect that realization comes of the number of union, fraternal, lodges, dances and social gatherings take place every night in the public halls of the city. On an average, ten union meetings are held in the Labor Temple every night and the Longshoremen and two or three other unions have meeting places elsewhere.

The business of the unions is not expected to be particularly injured by the inability to call the members together in meeting. All of them have their agents and executives who have power to deal with a good many questions which arise and they do not expect that the closing order will last long enough to interfere with the conduct of some of the major problems that come up.

The loss to the lessees of halls and theatres will be most serious, because it comes at a period of the year when they have to derive enough revenue to carry them through the slack seasons. The summer time constitutes the lean time for the lessees and owners of halls, and they are not able to save much on the expense side. The prin[...]

The Vancouver Daily Sun *ran this explanation of a "closed town" on the front page, October 19, 1918.*

Courier killed two birds with one stone in its advice column on how to avoid the 'flu and at the same time take the Victory Bond campaign over the top: "Use camphor, quinine and courage — buy Victory Bonds; Keep your feet warm — on the first symptom of 'cold feet' — buy Victory Bonds." As the epidemic seemed to be on the wane, it was planned to reopen the churches and schools on November 10, but the return to normal had to be postponed when an outbreak appeared in Chinatown. The area was placed under quarantine and an isolation hospital was set up in the old Lum Lock residence on Ellis Street. A superstition reported to exist among the Chinese of the city was noted on November 14: "... an evil spirit, which had taken upon itself the guise of a young white boy of about six years of age. The spirit seemed to be somewhat timid, and lurked around outbuildings and yards, keeping away from lighted stores and dwellings. It only appeared after dark, but that it exists and had been seen there was not the slightest doubt, to the Chinese. The spirit wears no shoes or stockings, and all who have seen it have been afflicted with the new disease and had [sic] died ..."

Sylvia Harper Cummings, telephone agent at Salmon Arm, lived at the back of the office so she could take night calls. During the epidemic the telephones rang constantly, often when there were no lines available at all. When she got 'flu herself, she rigged up an extension at her bedside and carried on with the job.

Kamloops was stricken on October 11; eight days later there were twenty-two cases and two deaths. Schools were closed, and public meetings banned. The hospital, built in 1912, could not handle all the cases, so emergency facilities were set up at the barracks for Indian patients and at the Patricia Hotel for whites. Influenza returned to Kamloops mildly in 1919, but so seriously in 1920 that the ban on public meetings had to be revived for three weeks.

By mid-October the first deaths had occurred at Prince Rupert, and Mayor McClymont appealed to the public for spare beds to be used at the Salvation Army citadel and the Borden Street school. Ten co-workers of a Hindu man who died in Prince Rupert cremated his body on a pyre at the Fairview Cemetery.

A New Westminster boy, Paul Monahan, was one of sixty students sent home by the Oblate Fathers when St. John's College in Edmonton was closed. The train on which fifteen-year-old Paul was riding struck a snow slide in the Rockies and was stalled without heat for nine hours. The boys got off and enjoyed a snowball fight, but when Monahan got home he had influenza and was kept in bed for four weeks. Later, when his mother told him he hadn't said a word in all that time, he could only shake his head. "I must have been really sick!"

/ E.A. Rosoman, who was born at Grindrod, British Columbia, was taken to a Victoria hospital at the age of three for surgery. Hardly through the operation, he contracted 'flu — as did almost all the nurses. His father, just returned from the war, was at a military hospital in Esquimault, and his mother came to the hospital to help the over-worked nurses with the child's care. She was taken sick herself and had to leave. "An army veteran in the next bed took over my care for the next ten days until my mother was well enough to return. I have wanted hundreds of times to know the name of that man and to thank him. Without his help I probably wouldn't be here today."

Influenza had reached Victoria early in October, and public meetings were banned from the eighth of that month until the twentieth day of November. To relieve the pressure on city hospitals, the old fire hall on Kingston Street, the Fairfield fire hall at Five Points, and a residence at 1124 Fort Street were fitted out as emergency hospitals; the military took over buildings at Stadacona Park when facilities at the Willows camp became overcrowded. The Pantages Theatre closed its doors, as did other public buildings. Girls were advised to stop kissing their sailor friends.

An English girl, too young to get into the nursing program at home, came to Canada to wait out the time. (In the end, she married here and never did go back to England.) When she answered the call for volunteers, she was assigned to one of the big emergency hospitals where she cared for men who had been brought in, sick, from the ships. One patient tried everyone's ingenuity; he wouldn't stay in bed. Finally, in desperation, the volunteer pinned him into his bedclothes with the large safety pins used for kilts, but in no time at all he was up and walking around the halls with his mattress on his back.

Vancouver's first case was reported on October 5, and when the epidemic was at last considered over in the following spring, it had taken the lives of 981 residents. St. Paul's and Vancouver

General hospitals were soon overcrowded, and the University of British Columbia auditorium, King Edward High School, and south Vancouver's Selkirk school were taken over for emergency accommodation. Even those added beds didn't prove to be enough, and a temporary building accommodating two hundred more beds was erected in less than three weeks at Twelfth and Heather.

Dr. Harry Milburn looked back on those busy days at King Edward School: "I remember those big rooms with those windows 'way up high and the rows of cots, and the nurses, white-attired with white masks, attending them. They looked like ghosts walking through a graveyard."

One Vancouver man who obeyed orders to the letter went straight to bed when he felt ill — still clad in overalls and boots. Severe depression was reported among some of the patients, and one, a rancher living on Malcolm Island, committed suicide.

Mical Olsen, who arrived in Vancouver as a ship's officer on a Norwegian vessel in 1907, was by 1918 the captain of a Hastings Mill tug boat towing logs from higher up the British Columbia coast to a Vancouver sawmill. The work was hard, and conditions on the boats were not very comfortable. When the men got wet there was neither time nor space to dry off, and of course many of them got 'flu. They availed themselves of liquor available by prescription from Vancouver doctors. The prescriptions cost two dollars each. The government liquor store had been opened for three hours on Sunday, October 20; the city's supply of camphor would be exhausted in two or three days; and "cinnamon and other anti-influenzal drugs" were running short, a newspaper noted.

Finally, on November 18, Victoria's ban on public gatherings was lifted, and the following day the city of Vancouver and the lower mainland followed suit.

THE NORTH

Just as it had on the Labrador coast, the 'flu slashed its way across the rest of the north. It attacked a highly vulnerable population with devastating force, sometimes totally destroying Indian and Eskimo settlements and hunting camps where the people, far from medical help, were quite unable to fight back on their own. The Indians, who were said to have a miraculous ability to recover from serious physical injury, lacked any defenses against respiratory infections.

At Beaver Indian Reserve, near what is now the town of Fairview, Alberta in the Peace River area, some 85 percent of the people, who lived in tiny log cabins or wigwams, died between November 1918 and April 1919. Traditionally, each successful hunter shared a big feed with his fellows, so there was no stored food to draw on during the epidemic. Sick men went out in a desperate attempt to catch a rabbit — or anything at all — and often didn't make it back. The Indian agent, who lived fifteen or twenty miles from the reserve, was sick himself and couldn't help. There were not enough strong people left to put the dead bodies up on roofs to keep the dogs from consuming them.

Dr. O.D. Weeks of Calgary, who volunteered to help the Cree Indians in the Fort McMurray and Lac La Biche areas of northern Alberta, found them in dire straits, huddled together "in fear, and in sympathy," with the dead and the dying all together. At one cabin he found a delirious woman on the floor, clutching an eight-month-old baby who had been dead for forty-eight hours. "The woman protested strongly when the child was taken away," reported the *Edmonton Bulletin*. At another cabin a woman and three children were ill. Also in the cabin was a baby two-and-one-half weeks old, unwashed and untended since its birth. At the home of the chief at Beaver Lake Reserve seven people lay on the floor, all dead except the chief himself.

At Big Bay there were at least twenty bodies unburied, stored in a vacant cabin, with no-one strong enough to dig their graves. Dr. Weeks, a strong supporter of inoculation, pointed out that at one Indian mission where there were fifty children, five adult sisters, and one priest, all of whom had been inoculated, none had contracted the disease even though it was all around them. He credited his own ability to keep going night and day to taking weekly inoculations against the germ.

One Alberta provincial police patrol from Edson, west of Edmonton, found four dead in a tepee twenty miles from the town. Surviving were a woman and an infant child, both in a critical state. Shortly after his arrival the woman died. He buried the dead people and carried the infant, wrapped in blankets, back to Edson, where he eventually found it a foster home.

In 1918 Brother Frederick Leach, OMI, taught at the mission school at Berens River on the northeastern shores of Lake Winnipeg. During freeze-up and break-up the little community was isolated, so the arrival of the passenger steamer *Wolverine* at the end of October, making its last trip for the year, was an important event. The residents heard that some of the crew were sick but paid little attention until, three days later, all but a few of them were ill. There were no cures. Two men of the cloth who remained well, Father Valès and the Methodist minister the Reverend Percy Jones, did all they could to give physical care and spiritual consolation. Every day the people lying ill heard the distressing sound of gun shots — the method adopted to announce that someone had died.

Diaries from the isolated Hudson's Bay posts remain to record the dreary events. At York Factory, Manitoba, the 'flu began in October; by February, with the temperature at forty degrees below zero, the report reads laconically: "Quite a lot of York people laid up." In March, Indians passing by Shamattawa chopped wood and visited the fishing nets of the sick people, and when they reported to the post what they had found, a dog train of provisions and medicines was sent. More 'flu was reported at Crooked Bank and Sturgeon Lake. Not surprisingly, little business was being done at the York Factory store.

Fort Alexander, Manitoba, November 7, 1918: "The Spanish 'flu has a firm hold on everybody here and we are not allowing anyone in the store or house but are serving them from the doorway as a precaution against us getting it." Despite this vigilance, by January 6, 1919 all residents but one had caught the disease and there had been forty-three deaths.

Cyril Chaboyeur remembers when the 'flu began at Cumberland House in northern Saskatchewan: "People living along the lake saw the darkness coming from the north. As soon as the darkness came here people started to fall down." Infant Nancy Thomas, six months old, crawled around the floor crying for food and attention as her mother lay ill, unable to help her or even call out. The Hudson's Bay Company diary began to report 'flu in November 1918, continuing through December and January. On February 6, 1919 it ran: "Working at coffins and getting wood. No time for anything else. Dismal times." Reports of illness and death came to the post from Montreal Lake, Pine Bluffs, The Landing, Sturgeon Lake, Birch River, Budd's Point, Brave Lake, and The Pas.

In 1919 Joseph MacAuley, whose grandfather John Richard Settee was the second native Anglican minister at Cumberland House, came home after serving in the army. He arrived three days after his brother Dan had died of 'flu. "There were no doctors there but there was a nurse, the wife of an RNWMP man. She tried to get the people something to eat. She pulled dead bodies to the church on a hand sleigh because with everyone sick there was nobody to bury them until spring." Dogs, frantic with hunger, broke into the building and chewed at the bodies. In mid-February Constable Paquette of the RNWMP brought two nurses from The Pas. Chaboyeur remembers that they gave people soup to drink, but nothing seemed to help. "If you got sick, you died."

In the end the epidemic virtually wiped out the reserve, which was situated about three miles from the town of Cumberland House, and the people who were left moved to Pine Bluffs and Budd Springs. Eventually they returned to the old reserve, and descendants of the 'flu dead now take care of the graveyard. In 1962 a memorial service was held where the old church had stood.

The Reverend Adam Cuthand, then five years old, lived with his family at the Cree Little Pine Reserve along the Battle River in Saskatchewan. The 'flu hit heavily on the reserve, especially among the people who lived in tents. The Cuthand family, who had cattle and a large garden, lived in a warm house formerly used as a teacherage, but even so Adam caught the disease and his younger sister died of it. The two hundred people on the reserve were discouraged, despondent, without hope, until word came from the Hobbema Reserve in Alberta, "perhaps by mail, perhaps by moccasin telegraph [by word of mouth]." Someone there had had a dream telling the people to dance, to hold a pow-wow. At Little Pine they began with a feast and prayers, then held a dance. "It raised the morale of the people," Cuthand says.

The Hudson's Bay post at Ile-à-la-Crosse, Saskatchewan, reported in November that there was 'flu there and at Green Lake. It was bad at Cold Lake with twenty adults dead, and at Canoe

Lake nearly all were down with 'flu. At church on Sunday, December 15, at Ile-à-la-Crosse there were very few people and all were coughing. More reports came from Old Souris, La Ronge, and Pine River, all equally discouraging. By January 1919 there was sickness at Clear Lake, Big River, English River, and Wapachanack.

And so the dreary reports continued. Flu, and more 'flu.

The Department of Indian Affairs summed up for the year ending March 31, 1919: "The Indians of Ontario in common with other sections of the population suffered very severely from the epidemic of influenza and the mortality among them as a result of this cause was high. The Department's medical officers and the agency staffs spared no effort in their efficient and energetic efforts to prevent the spread of the disease. Unfortunately it was impossible to secure adequate medical attention for the Indians living in the more outlying parts, a circumstance which is not surprising in view of the fact that a similar situation existed in the majority of the white communities throughout the Dominion."

Nova Scotia Indians, the report said, had experienced a lesser percentage of deaths as a result of the influenza epidemic than had the whites of the province, but had also suffered an outbreak of smallpox. On Prince Edward Island, only three deaths directly due to influenza were reported among the Indian population. Indians in Saskatchewan suffered a very heavy mortality from influenza and "many of them have been left in a very delicate state of health as a result thereof. In some localities it was accompanied by a form of bronchial pneumonia of a virulent nature." In British Columbia, influenza was particularly serious among the people of the Kamloops and Lytton bands. "The disease was particularly hard on the aged and those of weak lungs. Several chiefs were among the victims. Industrially it interfered with the saving of the root crops, and in several instances fields of potatoes were left with the tubers in the ground, because so many were sick that there were none left who were well enough to dig them," the report said.

The year of 1920 saw the 'flu strike at Lac La Ronge. Harold Kemp, later to be collector of Customs and Excise for the Port of Prince Albert, found himself along with two friends acting as cook, choreboy, nurse, and undertaker. They dosed the sick people with the only medications they had — hot lemonade and painkiller — and kept them warm. It was all they could do. The appreciation of their Indian patients was touching. "While we tended these people, nursed them with our pitiful efforts, we heard no word of complaint, no suggestion of self-pity. They were so grateful for what we were able to do, and if any worry or anxiety were expressed, it was not for themselves but for their friends and relatives. And when, to many of them, came the consciousness that they were beyond our help, they accepted the fact with quiet resignation."

With the ground frozen too hard to dig, the three men had to store the bodies of the dead in the icy church. They sent messages for help by departing freighter, but got no response. After three weeks their meagre supply of medication was at an end so one of the men set out for Prince Albert with a special team of five good dogs, hoping to cover the two hundred miles in three days. At Montreal Lake he was lucky enough to get a team of horses, which speeded his trip, and less than a week later Lac La Ronge had the services of a doctor, a nurse, and a mounted policeman.

But in the meantime, the two left behind had faced a tough task. With the help of the Reverend Mr. Hives, the local minister, who by now had recovered from his own illness, and two other men who had also recovered, they checked nearby camps. In a cabin at one of the camps they found a dead man, a dead woman, and one still-living woman and her child. In one bunk was a man whose mind had snapped with the horror he had seen. They loaded the living people onto sleighs and toboggans and removed the dead bodies in order to burn the cabin so that they could dig a grave in the thawed ground beneath. One of them came up with the suggestion that they return the dead bodies to the cabin and cremate them, but this idea was met with a flat "No" from the minister. His word prevailed. They followed their original plan, and, when the burial had been accomplished, Mr. Hives read the Burial Service.

Meanwhile at Stanley, on the Churchill River, a trader for Revillon Frères was fighting the epidemic almost single-handed. To solve the problem of graves for the score of people who had died, he used a shallow mine shaft in which he placed the dead upright, "facing the east, looking for the Dawn."

Marcel Chappius, who had served with the Royal North West Mounted Police at Ile-à-la-Crosse during the epidemic there, was to see the 'flu strike yet again. In 1921, a year after the name of the force had been changed to the Royal Canadian Mounted Police, he was transferred to the Fond du Lac detachment at the east end of Lake Athabasca, south of the border between Saskatchewan and the Northwest Territories. Just before Easter in 1922, the disease struck down the native people who were in the habit of coming to the Roman Catholic Mission at Fond du Lac for Mass at Christmas, Easter, and in July. On their way in from their camps, sometimes hundreds of miles away, they travelled night and day; people sickened, and many of the old ones died. The remainder continued their journey, leaving the dead at camps along the way. Chappius and his assistant followed the trails back as best they could and found nearly eighty bodies. The policemen tied the bodies to a toboggan, two or three at a time, and made the laborious journey back with them to Fond du Lac, where they found the priest ill and unable to conduct the burial service — and the ground frozen too hard to dig graves. The Hudson's Bay post had bales and bales of canvas duck, thirty inches wide, for sale for tents. Obtaining permission from the post manager, the two men used this canvas to sew a covering for each body and stacked them, like cordwood, in a warehouse.

When the weather started to warm up in May and the bodies began to thaw, there was fear of still another epidemic. The priest, still sick, gave permission to place the bodies all together in long trenches. The Indians who were still at the post were sent back to their camps so they could have the benefit of open air and avoid contact with people outside their own community. In July, when it was time for the summer mass, the Indians returned to Fond du Lac, and the priest, who by that time had recovered, conducted a communal burial service for all those who had died.

The middle of January 1919 saw the departure from Dawson, Yukon Territory, of a five-man party, including a native guide and trailbreaker, under the direction of the famed Arctic musher Staff Sgt. W.J.D. Dempster. The group, travelling by dogteam and carrying fifteen pounds of medical supplies, took twenty days to reach Fort McPherson in the Northwest Territories.

Through much of the north, there was 'flu all during the 1920s. At the Roman Catholic Mission in Brochet, Manitoba, it was Easter of 1922 when eleven people in a party returning to camp after Easter devotions sickened and died. There were deaths at the mission through April, May, and June; only three residents escaped the scourge. Father Egenolf recorded in his diary that it took an entire month for him to recover normal strength. Births at Brochet that year were twenty-two and deaths, thirty-one.

An outbreak at Coronation Gulf and Bathurst Inlet in 1926 took forty-three lives, and in 1927 another in the same areas killed thirty-one. Sgt. F. Anderton, the RCMP officer in charge at Cambridge Bay, reported early in January 1928 a further outbreak: "In the first place, the sickness has commenced after the arrival of the boats from the outside; this may have no material bearing on the cases, but it is a fact, I am stating it, and it has been my experience, both on the river and on the coast, the whole population of the settlements, white and native, do get colds after the arrival of the boat or ship.

"These colds do not seriously bother the white settlers, but they certainly do the natives, who are today partially wearing white man's clothes and partially native clothes. When they wear white men's clothes they do not wear sufficient to compensate for the clothing they have been used to all their lives, and it is no uncommon sight to see a native going around with fur pants on, and nothing above but a thin woollen undershirt, even though it may be raining at the time; when he gets cold towards evening, he puts on deerskins over the wet undershirt, which remains there and dries on his body; also when they wear white man's clothing, it remains on their bodies from the time it is procured until the time it rots off, and it is never changed or washed."

Discussing the serious concern about the lack of hygiene among the native people at that time, Sergeant Anderton said: "In the case of sickness spreading rapidly amongst them, I will simply state what happened with one native family here last fall, named Nuckahou, comprising the man, two wives and four children, seven in all. During the summer he built an igloo, of a layer of rock, then a layer of sod, also the sleeping platform was built of sod and rock; in the fall this igloo naturally drew dampness, and the inside was always wet. When they were all taken sick, he would not vacate it. I attended his family throughout their sickness; they were all lying on the platform, naked and covered by two blankets and three deerskins, and would not get out of bed for anything."

Archibald Lang Fleming, later to be the first Anglican bishop of the Arctic, went to the western Arctic for the first time in 1928 by an arduous route: by rail from Edmonton to the end of steel at Waterways on the Clearwater River, then 2,514 miles by paddle steamer on the Athabasca and Mackenzie rivers to the Arctic Ocean. At Fort Smith he boarded the *Distributor*, "a flat-bottomed wooden scow with two superimposed upper decks that looked very much like the verandahs of early Canadian and American houses." At Hay River, on the fourth day of July 1928, James and Sarah Simon, whom Fleming described as a "fine and handsome Loucheaux couple," boarded the *Distributor*; the Simons had been studying English at Hay River and were to accompany and help the then Archdeacon Fleming in his work at Fort McPherson.

Influenza broke out on the ship and at Fort Norman the Simons became ill. Sarah Simon, who lives now at Fort McPherson, remembers how sick their little girls were and that no-one knew what the disease was called.

In his autobiography Fleming recounts: "At each settlement after the steamer departed the people succumbed and the epidemic raged up and down the river, taking a final toll of more than 300 Indians." The air remained hot and stuffy, adding to the discomfort of the sick passengers and to the difficulties of Nurse McCabe, the only medical person on board. When they reached Fort McPherson, where the original fort had been erected in 1846, the archdeacon arranged for the Simons to move into the rectory. Sarah Simon remembered: "We are all sick in bed. A week later everybody got sick. No doctors, no nurses, we have only a little dispensary. Night and day the sick called James and Mr. Owen [a young man who had been there a year], and they went from tent to tent to have a prayer with them." At last two men who were not very sick were sent to Aklavik. They brought back an RCMP corporal and another man, who together turned the church into a hospital. The patients drank a tea made from wild berries, and a broth of fish.

Fleming went on to Aklavik where, he reports with enormous restraint, the government doctor "declined to stay and see us through and departed for the south on board the ship. We were left to battle against the epidemic as best we could. It was a sad business and our hearts went out to the Eskimo, the Indians and the half-breeds in their misery. They lay in their tents or in the cramped quarters of the boats with the passionless simplicity of sick children, too weak to attend to their own needs."

As had happened elsewhere, the people defied advice when they began to feel better. They went outside, caught a chill, and often within a few hours were carried off by pneumonia. With the ground frozen to nearly a foot beneath the surface, digging graves was an exhausting business; the dead were buried in blankets or skin sleeping bags.

/Mounted policemen rolled up their sleeves and went to work to try to alleviate the distressing conditions of the natives along the Arctic coast. Some of them moved into Eskimo communities to look after and feed the sick people, they fished and hunted, and they tended the dogs that were so vitally important to both the trappers and the traders/One of these men was Alcide Lamothe, a nineteen-year-old RCMP constable from Hull, Quebec who had been with the force for a year when he was transferred from Fairmont Barracks, E Division, in Vancouver, to Shingle Point on the Beaufort Sea. There he replaced Constable Bob Kells in the job of caring for the sick. Besides the members of the Hudson's Bay post, where Lamothe shared accommodation with the young English manager, there were about ten Eskimo families at Shingle Point. He found them lying sick, their coverings flung off. "Because of their high fevers they felt hot so they lay naked in the tents."

Shingle Point was a meeting place for the Eskimos, and the post was well supplied with canned and dried foodstuffs and some medicines. Lamothe took canned milk and soup to the sick people and, to supplement their diet, tried to catch fresh fish and animals. It was a bad year for hunting, however, and there was nothing to be had. "We even had to feed the dogs canned meat," he said.

Two white trappers came along and stayed to help Lamothe and the Hudson's Bay manager. Among them they buried the dead people, wrapped in skins, in shallow individual graves; they could dig down only about a foot before striking ice. About half the Eskimo population around Shingle Point died.

Many years later, when Lamothe was working in Ottawa, he stopped an Eskimo couple on the street to ask what part of the Arctic they came from. He was surprised and pleased when the woman recognized him; one of the survivors of the epidemic at Shingle Point, she had been a child in 1928 when he was there.

Bill Nevin, who served with the Royal Canadian Mounted Police at Herschel Island in the Beaufort Sea during the 1930s, sums up: "Those lovable people — the Eskimo — seemed to be completely vulnerable to illness of almost any kind, unlike white people who had built up an immunity. There seemed to be no degree of illness with them. I could always see the Eskimo in one of two states: very well, or ill and ready to die."

Professionals and Valiant Volunteers

Canadians, still reeling under the impact of their losses to the war, were now required to go that extra mile and help their neighbors, despite what one woman described as "an almost visible fear." In country places, farmers went to the edge of their properties every morning to check for signs of activity at the next house; if there wasn't smoke rising from the chimney, they went to investigate. A small Montreal girl, sent by her mother to deliver hot soup to the music teacher living alone in a rooming house, was instructed to go up the stairs and place the bowl just over the sill — not one step into the room.

Often it was an agonizing decision: go to the aid of friends and relatives, perhaps imperilling the safety of their own families, or keep away? The moral decision to close the doors was frequently as difficult as that to go out and help. Mrs. Burton Thomas Read of Upper Nappan, Nova Scotia, got word that her sister's baby was coming and help was needed, but because there was 'flu in the house no-one would come. Mrs. Read had a nursing infant herself, and her husband was away so could not be consulted. Finally, leaving her children in the care of the eldest, she hitched a horse to the driving carriage and drove to her sister's home.

At Bury, Quebec, the village undertaker was unable to keep pace with the work and called on his brother to help him. Carlos Stokes hesitated. He had four children, his wife was ill (although not with 'flu); should he take the risk? His wife decided for him. "Bring me that square of camphor and a thin handkerchief," she directed. She sewed the little package onto her husband's undershirt and sent him on his way. Neither he, nor any of his family, caught the 'flu.

Canada's doctors had gone to war. In British Columbia alone, two hundred had joined the services: there were few left at home to cope with the 'flu epidemic. Retired doctors rose to the challenge and, working side by side with those in practice, put in almost unbelievable hours, snatching a wink of sleep wherever they could between calls. They got around by whatever means was available — car, sleigh, horseback, bicycle, snowshoe, or Shank's mare. A medical team on Vancouver Island, using a forty-foot boat with a large one-cylinder engine, fought twenty-foot tides on their way to tend lumberjacks at Port McNeill, eighty-five miles up the coast. Weyburn, Saskatchewan doctors blessed the lack of winter snow because it meant they could get to their rural patients by car. All were not so lucky; at Lachute, Quebec and Montague, Prince Edward Island snow piled high and doctors had to travel by sleigh.

Overwhelmingly, Canadians who recall that terrible era remember their doctors with an affection and respect bordering on awe. "He worked to the point of exhaustion"; "He only catnapped"; "He had a driver and slept just between calls." Sometimes, sadly, the strain those doctors imposed upon themselves was too great and their health was permanently damaged. More than one hundred doctors died in Ontario and the prairie provinces alone. While preaching to their patients that it was essential to rest in bed even after they began to feel better, the men and women who tended them couldn't obey their own rules. There were so few of them, and so many sick people.

Ella Parsons, wife of a doctor in Red Deer, Alberta, wrote her mother on November 12, 1918 that she was deeply worried about the health of her over-worked husband. Just after writing the letter she got 'flu herself and died within days, leaving her sick sons in a room down the hall.

In Toronto Dr. Kenneth McLaren, bone-tired after more than a month of twenty-hour days followed by a hectic period in his own practice as convalescents struggled to regain their strength, was quite worn out by early summer. He spotted an ad in the paper for a cottage to rent in Georgian Bay for the month of July. To Dr. McLaren, its chief charm was that there could be no communication with the outside world. He signed the lease and for one whole luxurious month just rested, secure in the knowledge that no telephone could ring.

Dr. James Collins, who practiced at Vernon River, Prince Edward Island, kept his daughters almost as busy as he was himself, taking them with him on his calls and directing them to

A letter written by Mrs. Ella Parsons of Red Deer, Alberta just days before she died of 'flu. (Courtesy Dr. W.D. Parsons)

"sweep the floors, do the dishes; do whatever the family needs." As well as the quinine he prescribed, he had rum sent for the patients on the Murray Harbour train. Again, the girls were pressed into service to drive around and deliver the bottles to Elliottvale and Armdale. An exceptionally strong man who weighed three hundred pounds, he worked day and night. His daughter Mary, who later became a nurse, attributes his success to his kindness: "The office was packed all the time, and he lost only one patient."

Dr. A.T. Leatherbarrow of New Brunswick, who was with the Army Medical Corps in Saint John during 1918, recalled that it was not unusual to see twenty or thirty people sick in the morning and to find half of them dead by nightfall. "There wasn't enough staff left alive to administer treatment to anyone. It was a case of 'survive yourself, or die.' " Luckily he seemed to have had an immunity and was able to work constantly throughout the epidemic, but he knows that hundreds died without ever seeing a doctor.

A Prince Rupert, British Columbia doctor was so tired that he fell asleep at the wheel of his car and drove it off a cliff. Fortunately, the car landed upright and he was unhurt.

Sometimes it seemed to the doctors that there wasn't much they could do for the patients when they did see them. Dr. Elizabeth Bagshaw, who practiced in Hamilton, Ontario until five years before her death at the age of 100 years, was one of the busiest doctors in the city. Her first 'flu case was a woman from London, Ontario on her way home from New York; she became ill in Hamilton and died there. "The worst problem we had was with pregnant women," Dr. Bagshaw said. "They usually miscarried and nearly always died."

A quarter of the Hamilton doctors were ill themselves, and the rest closed their offices so people would not gather and pass the germ around. Dr. Bagshaw made more than twenty house calls a day. "We had nothing to give them as injections, Aspirin was almost the only thing." Eventually she got 'flu herself, although luckily she recovered after only a few days in bed. As well as her patient load, she had to tend visiting relatives who were ill and another woman doctor who had no-one to look after her. "I brought her to my house and somehow we all looked after each other. We were so weak that when we carried tea upstairs we didn't bother with a saucer because that would have been extra weight to carry." They craved odd things to eat as they were recuperating. Dr. Bagshaw wanted celery, and only celery.

In September 1918 Godfrey Bird and his brother Edward set out with their parents to drive from Gananoque, Ontario, near Kingston, to attend medical school in Toronto. Although they were only seventeen and sixteen it would be their second year; only junior matriculation was required to begin the course. With their father a doctor and their mother a nurse, neither of the boys had considered any career but medicine.

The roads were poor and the travelling tiring. They all wore goggles, caps, and dusters, and they went to bed with unwashed faces in order not to irritate already wind-burned skin. Even the direct route of one hundred and eighty miles took two days to drive in 1918, and that year Dr. and Mrs. Bird elected to take the long way around, going south of Lake Ontario and through the United States, making it an even longer journey. During a stopover at Rochester, New York, the family attended a vaudeville theatre where a warning of 'flu was made from the stage and local patrons wore gauze masks.

In Toronto the boys settled into their lodgings and registered for classes, but within two weeks the college was closed because of 'flu, and they received word to go home by train to help their father.

It was a gruelling world they entered back in Gananoque. Dr. James McCammon came out of retirement to help Dr. Bird in the emergency. Godfrey was assigned to drive one doctor, and Edward, the other. Godfrey Bird, now retired from medical practice in Gananoque, recalls: /"We would start off in the morning with twenty or more calls to make, both in town and in the country, and everywhere we would overtake or meet a funeral. My father found people curled up in bed, highly feverish and without hope. He propped them up on pillows so their lungs could clear. I attribute his remarkable success with this dreadful illness, for which there was no specific cure, to his appearance of confidence and the hope he inspired."/

After morning rounds Dr. Bird and his sons went home for lunch. As they sat at the dining room table the doctor dictated prescriptions to his sons, and Mrs. Bird dispensed the medicines to people lined up on the walk leading to the office door at the side of the house. When afternoon office hours began, she stood at the door of the waiting room with a thermometer in one hand and a pad of paper in the other, recording temperatures and pulse rates to save her husband time. Most people still preferred to take salicylates (aspirin) dissolved in colored water, rather than in the recently-introduced tablet form.

From a normal patient load of twenty-three to twenty-six people a day, Dr. Bird's Day Book shows an increase at the height of the epidemic to eighty or ninety persons. On October 12 he paid fifty-eight house calls and six days later, Drs. Bird and McCammon together called on seventy-five patients at their homes. By November 11 the house calls had dropped to nine a day, and by the eighteenth, to six. The epidemic was on the wane in Gananoque.

In later years, Dr. Bird Sr. often spoke to his sons of the bravery of the women in the community, many sick to death with worry about their own families. "Still, they went out to help someone else."

At the farming village of Upper Windsor, New Brunswick, cars were put away in winter. Snow ploughs, built of heavy planks in the form of a wing and pulled by three or four teams of horses, cleared only enough snow for the passage of one horse-drawn sleigh. When two met on the road, one driver had to pull into a neighbor's driveway to allow the other to pass.

During the winter of 1918, when the 'flu struck at Upper Windsor, George E. Robinson pulled a hand sled about two miles along the road through the village to deliver mail and groceries from Wilson's store to the stricken families, and to take them nourishing soups made by his wife. Verna Robinson Prosser, who was ten years old, remembers: "Grandmother's soup kettle was never off the stove. She made big pots of chicken and beef soup, and poured it into smaller kettles for Grandfather to deliver to the sick people. They would put the empty kettle from the day before on the step, and he would bring that back to be filled again."

There was a very occasional sour note in the picture of self-sacrifice. Some Vancouver pharmacists raised the price of camphor from 40 cents to $6.50 a pound in one week, and in Saskatchewan a doctor charged $35.00 to disinfect a seven-room house. In Calgary, a group of young women posed as professional nurses and charged patients $25.00 a day for their "services," at a time when private nurses in Montreal, who worked around the clock with five hours off during the afternoon, were getting $2.00. Later, when Montreal nurses discussed raising their fees to $3.00, people said: "They'll never get it, they're pricing themselves out of the market."

With 2,400 Canadian nurses serving overseas and another 500 on duty at military hospitals here, there were few left to tend the civilian population. In Vancouver so many nurses had gone to war that, in 1918, there were only 200 RNs on the roster, and by 1919 the number had dropped to 125 because so many were ill themselves or were nursing their own families.

Buildings everywhere were commandeered as temporary hospitals. The auditorium at the University at British Columbia was one, and the Jockey Club in Hamilton another. Schools, being closed anyway, were logical choices; in small towns the hotel was often used. Churches with basement kitchens for congregational dinners turned them over to volunteers, who cooked up strengthening foods for other volunteers to deliver to sick people. Dorothea Galley Inkster, a teacher at King Edward School in Toronto, volunteered her services at the kitchens of the Central Technical School on Harbord Street. The workers cut beef into little cubes, boiled it, and put it into Gem jars. In another room they made chocolate syrup to be mixed with milk, and in still another area mixed orange and whites of egg.

In Hamilton, Ontario one hundred and fifty members of the IODE used the kitchen of the First Methodist Church to prepare food for the sick. For eleven weeks, Sundays and Christmas Day included, they provided an average of eleven hundred meals per day. "The money to buy the many tons of food supplies used was freely contributed, often coming in large sums from unknown sources. Medical men freely expressed the opinion that this service did more to overcome the epidemic than anything else," a church history recounts.

With schools closed, teachers came forward by the thousands to help out. One such volunteer was Ethel Dickinson, a domestic science teacher in St. John's, Newfoundland, who had gone to England in 1915 to visit her aunt and had stayed on to serve as a volunteer nurse in military hospitals. She returned to St. John's in the summer of 1918 to resume her teaching career, but when the schools closed for the epidemic, she turned again to nursing the sick. In October, while working at the Seamen's Institute, she caught the disease herself and died two days later, at the age of thirty-eight.

So great was the affection for Ethel Dickinson that the people of St. John's contributed four thousand dollars for a gray Aberdeen granite monument to her memory. Still standing in Cavendish Square, where it was dedicated by Governor Harris on the second anniversary of her death, the cross bears this inscription: "This shaft, surmounted by the world emblem of sacrifice, is set up by a grateful public in memory of Ethel Dickinson, volunteer nurse, who in the great epidemic of 1918 gave her life while tending patients at King George V Institute [the Seamen's Institute], St. John's."

Another teacher who gave her life during the epidemic was Eleanor Beaubier, who was teaching in southeastern Saskatchewan. Instead of returning to her Manitoba home when the school closed, she went from house to house to nurse the sick, finally having them all moved to a large house where the doctor could visit everyone at once. Some of the surviving settlers believed she was successful because of the strength of her will: "She just would not allow people to die." Finally, exhausted and weakened, she caught the disease and died at the age of twenty-four, despite the ministrations of a trained nurse and four doctors — and the prayers of the community. The people never forgot her, and in 1927 the village was renamed Beaubier in her memory.

Other communities also showed their gratitude to those teachers who stepped into the breach. In Kamloops, British Columbia, the school board voted that teachers should receive their salaries as usual even though the schools had been closed for two months; the same was done in Prince Edward Island, and the Saskatchewan government voted to continue grants to all the schools.

Despite the number of St. John Ambulance instructors serving overseas with the Army Medical Corps, the organization did not lose sight of its original goal, the instruction of the civilian population. Between 1914 and 1919, more than sixty thousand Canadians took those courses in first aid and home nursing, and during the epidemic the graduates not only nursed the sick but cleaned their houses and chopped wood as well. In several small

Ontario hospitals, with every staff member sick, the VADs (girls and women who belonged to the Voluntary Aid Detachment of St. John Ambulance) found themselves in charge. In Saskatoon the wife of the St. John Ambulance president, Mrs. C.L. Drurie, caught 'flu and died while nursing at the temporary hospital.

On October 24, an Edmonton newspaper published this notice: "An Appeal to All! Do not hesitate — you are needed. Telephone

ONTARIO EMERGENCY VOLUNTEER
HEALTH AUXILIARY

WANTED—VOLUNTEERS!!

The Provincial Board of Health, with the authority of the Government of Ontario, has organized an "Ontario Emergency Volunteer Health Auxiliary" for the purpose of training and supplying nursing help to be utilized wherever needed in combating the Influenza outbreak. A strong Executive has been formed in Toronto. It is recommended that each Municipal Council and Local Board of Health, working in co-operation, take immediate steps to form a local branch of this organization. The Volunteer Nurses will wear the officially authorized badge, "Ontario S.O.S." (Sisters of Service). This "S.O.S." call may be urgent. Classes taking lectures are already opened in the Parliament Buildings, Toronto (Private Bills Committee Room, ground floor), where they will be carried on every day at 10 a.m. and 3 p.m. until further notice. Young women of education are urged to avail themselves of this unique opportunity to be of real service to the community. If they are not needed, so much the better. If they are needed, we hope to have them ready. All towns and cities are urged to organize and prepare in a similar manner.

A Syllabus of Lectures is being sent to the Medical Officer of Health of all cities and towns. Further information may be had on application to John W. S McCullough, M.D., Chairman of Executive, Parliament Buildings, Toronto, Telephone Main 5800.

C. S. NEWTON, Sec.-Treas   W. D. McPHERSON, President.

J. W. S. McCULLOUGH, Chairman of Executive Committee.

Ontario training courses for volunteer nurses were advertised in the Toronto Daily Star *of October 15, 1918. (Photo courtesy Metropolitan Toronto Library Board)* your name to the St. John Ambulance Brigade, 31239." In Ontario, the provincial board of health organized the training of volunteer nurses under the name "Sisters of Service," abbreviated to SOS, with instruction by Dr. C.J. Copp of St. John Ambulance, and Dr. Margaret Patterson. The SOS was immediately organized in other areas of the province as well, and "To Young Lady Volunteers," the text of the lectures, was published in the *Globe*. On the west coast, St. John Ambulance workers responded to an appeal from C.C. Perry, Indian agent, to help nurse the Indians of Port Simpson and Metlakatla at the Salvation Army building in Prince Rupert, British Columbia.

Gertrude Murphy Charters, who had been teaching at Carmangay, Alberta, went home to Calgary when her school closed. She held a VAD certificate and had worked for a few days doing odd jobs for hard-pressed nurses at the General Hospital, but never had an opportunity to do any actual nursing. On October 2, a telephone call at four o'clock in the morning from her VAD supervisor changed all that. She was needed at the desperately hard-hit town of Drumheller. Her supervisor told her that one of her friends and a registered nurse would also be going. Five hours later, over the worried protests of her mother, she was on the train to Drumheller. All around her were passengers wearing gauze masks, but there was no friend and no nurse anywhere to be seen. She later discovered that her friend had come down with 'flu that morning, as had the nurse's husband. "Had I known I was going alone I never would have gone and I would have missed the most rewarding experience of my life," Gertrude Murphy Charters said later.

Although Drumheller was quarantined, because of her mission she was allowed to get off at the station. Other passengers had peered curiously at her uniform and had avoided passing her seat. "I got my first taste then of that paralyzing mass fear that was following the influenza epidemic around the world."

At the temporary hospital in the school, Gertrude Charters found herself all alone, with no nursing experience, in charge of twenty very ill men lying on back-breakingly low Winnipeg couches.* She bathed the hot faces and fed each man warm soup

---

*Low, narrow, coil-spring couches with sides that lifted up to make a double bed.

brought in from a restaurant. Volunteers brought in more men from the coal mines and carried out the bodies of those who had died. It became like a blur. Immigrants from Rumania, Poland, Austria, Italy, Hungary, far from home and frightened, in their delirium raved in their native tongues. Some thought the disease they had was the Black Death. "It's fear that's killing a lot of them. They won't fight it. They just give in — and die," Dr. Green said when he stopped to see them. Ill himself, he continued his rounds in a town that was literally filled with 'flu.

The night shift of volunteers came in at nine o'clock and by midnight, dizzy with fatigue, Gertrude Charters went at last to sleep at the home of one of the volunteers. His wife, just convalescing from 'flu herself, offered a warm welcome and a comfortable guest room to the weary girl.

Next morning, when she returned to what had been dubbed "The Wild Man's Ward" because so many of the sick men, determined to run away, had had to be strapped to their beds, she found that six had died in the night.

At last Red Cross supplies arrived and, best of all, a registered nurse who took onto her shoulders the burden of responsibility.

A month after Gertrude Murphy Charters had begun her demanding task the picture was beginning to brighten, but there were still eighty-four men and twenty-three women and children sick, as well as a further thirty convalescing.

After the epidemic had spent itself in Drumheller, Milton C. Switzer, the town druggist, was asked to try to straighten out the statistics. It was an impossible task. Although the patients' names had been attached to their beds when they were brought in, many of them had got up and wandered in their delirium. Sometimes they fell into someone else's bed, with another name tag on it, and if they died there, no-one knew who they were.

Yet another grim discovery awaited the authorities in Drumheller. Many of the European miners, bent on saving money, perhaps to bring their families to Canada, had dug caves into the sidehills for dwellings. Some who sickened there and died were not found until long after.

When the epidemic struck at Stratford, Ontario the Sisters of Loretto sent their boarders home and on a Saturday opened the convent as an emergency hospital. By Monday every bed was occupied by patients of all denominations, and the nuns had little time to rest until the emergency was over. One of them, in her detailed account of their sad, and happy, experiences, described their working garb: "We wore white night gowns over habits and masks. We were sights. You ought to see Mother Mary Eucheria with nightgown back to front."

A local woman who was bringing jellies for the patients was afraid of the 'flu but was reassured by a friend that the nuns were very careful and had soaked the curtains in Creoline. "See, there is the curtain," her friend said as they opened the door, but the curtain walked away; it was Mother Mary Eucheria in her back-to-front nightgown.

The city provided the convent with free coal, and cancelled gas, electric light, and water bills while the temporary hospital was in operation; townspeople, both Catholic and Protestant, helped with food and cleaning chores. The undertaker said this work had done more for the Loretto nuns than their forty years of teaching in the city. "No reward for teachers in this world. I hope it is not so in Heaven," the diarist commented.

When it was all over, the "nurses" were presented with a medal by the City of Stratford for their work in caring for the 'flu victims.

With the 'flu raging all over the continent, indeed all over the world, people lent a hand wherever they were. Beth Pears Dearden of the Toronto brick-making family, and granddaughter of Will Tattle, who owned a market garden where prestigious Forest Hills Village now stands, had taken a first-aid and home-nursing course from a St. John Ambulance instructor. When, at twenty, she was asked by her uncle in Hannah, North Dakota, to help him with the office work of his grain elevator business, she took her gray VAD uniform with its stiff white collar and cuffs with her — just in case. For ten dollars she bought a ticket on the train to Winnipeg, then continued by milk train to Snowflake, Manitoba and down into North Dakota, where her uncle met her and drove her home in his Overland touring car.

Soon after she arrived, in October 1918, she began to receive letters from her mother in Toronto warning her about the 'flu. Before long, it struck Hannah, and Beth wanted to help. "Although I wasn't a nurse, I did know a little about home nursing." A woman in the community, who already had two small children and was expecting twins, was desperately ill with 'flu. In the attic of the house lay the woman's husband and the two young children, all sick.

Neighbors were taking turns nursing the stricken family, and Beth volunteered to take the night shift. Mostly, her job was to keep the wood-stove well stoked up and to give the patients tea and soup. It was sixty degrees below zero in North Dakota that winter, so fire-tending was vitally important. "In my room at my uncle's home, a good strong house with a good furnace, in the mornings there was an inch of frost standing out like whiskers on the window panes," she remembers.

With small children of their own, her aunt and uncle were worried about Beth bringing infection into their house. "It was so cold in the back kitchen, where we entered, that I couldn't possibly have had a bath there without freezing to death. They passed out a tub of hot water; I put a few drops of crude carbolic into the water, sponged my hands and face and wiped my shoes, then changed into my regular clothing. I dropped my uniform into the tub before entering the house and it froze solid." The next night when she went back to the neighbor's house she wore a smock, not having a second uniform, and not until the emergency was over was her uniform thawed and properly washed.

For two nights Beth Dearden nursed the sick woman, taking over from the daytime helpers after her regular day's work, with no sleep except for occasional catnaps. When a replacement was found and Beth returned to the routine of office work, she was exhausted but satisfied; all her patients, even the pregnant woman, were on the road to recovery. Neither she nor anyone in her uncle's family got the infection, and the twin babies arrived safely. The mother, father, two children, and twins all survived.

In Alberta, the Women's Institute sponsored home-nursing and first-aid courses in fifty-four centres, and trained more than thirty-four hundred volunteers. Toronto ministers appealed for volunteers, and organizations such as the Imperial Order Daughters of the Empire, the Women's Canadian Club, the Graduate Nurses' Association, the Women's Conservative Club, the Women's Liberal Club, and the YWCA rose to the challenge.

In Ottawa, where on October 14 all stores except fruit, confectionery, stationery, book, and drugstores were instructed to close at 4:00 P.M., Mayor Harold Fisher made this appeal to the public: "I want to make it absolutely clear that people are dying in our midst because they are not provided with proper care. They are not dying because we do not know about them. We know where they are, but we have nobody to send. Knitting socks for soldiers is very useful work but we are now asking the women of Ottawa to get in the trenches themselves."

Policemen and firemen carried food and fuel into Montreal homes, and in Toronto ten thousand cards were given to postmen to distribute on their routes to get information on people who needed help.

A telegram went out to all offices of the Victorian Order of Nurses instructing them to disregard the clause in their charter that forbade the nursing of infectious cases. The chief superintendent's report for 1918 noted that because of the number of nurses who had gone overseas to serve, their ranks were sadly depleted, and those who remained had to make superhuman efforts to handle the work. The nurses had felt that the end of the war would bring the situation back to normal; instead they found themselves ". . . in the grip of a great epidemic as world-wide as the war and much more disastrous in its results on the life of the nation."

In Vancouver the VON published an appeal to persons living near the Florence Nightingale Home at the corner of Venables and Clark to provide rooms and breakfasts for volunteer nurses, adding that anyone who had previously had influenza in their homes could fearlessly provide this service.

In the magazine the *War Cry*, William J. Richards, commissioner of the Salvation Army, issued a call to all Salvationists to give every possible assistance to those who needed help. All across the country they rose magnificently to the occasion, nursing, cleaning, buying and cooking food, even laying out bodies for burial. In Toronto, an old man, asking for further help, praised the Salvation Army volunteers: "Send them two young ladies what was here yesterday," he requested. "They was the Army girls and they was so lovely and kind." As well as the practical work of nursing, they brought the comfort of prayer to the patients.

An editorial in the *War Cry* for October 26 exemplifies the practical approach for which the organization is famous: "There must be a complete trust in God and realization that whatever may happen to one in the course of one's duty will be in accordance with His will. . . . It would, in our opinion, be presumptuous to neglect any known precaution which it is possible to take and, at the same time, expect the protection of God. . . . To neglect to protect oneself in this case means danger to others because every person who neglects proper precautions spreads the infection wherever he or she goes."

Also active in alleviating the suffering of those stricken with 'flu was the Canadian Red Cross Society. Mrs. Shearwood of Montreal, a member of the Alberta Red Cross and honorary eastern Canadian purchasing agent for the branch, arranged a shipment of sheets, blankets, pillow cases, nurses' gowns, towels, and other supplies to the Red Cross provincial headquarters in Alberta. In Alberta, too, a Red Cross nurse went to the Pouce Coupe district where three thousand people were ill. Work done by a Red Cross nurse at Eastdale, on the outskirts of Toronto, led to the establishment of a permanent post of school nurse for the area.

The Reverend Leon B. Wright, then a student pastor at Pleasantville, Nova Scotia, left his duties to help care for the stricken people of the area. At the first home he found the mother was away in hospital and the father, two sons, and one daughter were all in bed with high temperatures. The grandfather, who was over ninety years old, was unable to do anything to help. The cows had not been milked, and none of the animals had been fed.

Mr. Wright summoned a neighbor's son to care for the livestock and set about doing what he could for the sick people. Local doctors, fearing that contamination might be spread through water, had recommended that soda be added to drinking water. "The sick man told me the soda might be in a glass jar in the food closet. I found something that looked right and took it to him. He agreed it was soda, so I mixed it with a glass of water and he drank it — but it came right back up.

"He said he didn't think it had been soda after all, so I asked the daughter. She was well enough by then to laugh. 'That's powdered borax,' she told me. So, that was my first medical nursing — washing out a stomach."

At another house he found the mother in very serious condition. He peeled and sliced onion into hot lard and tore clothing to make poultice covers. Coming into her room with the poultice ready, he found her gasping, choking for breath. Hastily, he mixed mustard with the hot lard still in the frying pan and wrapped a cloth soaked in the mixture around her throat. With the poultice on her chest and the compress in place, he got her into a sitting position with a chair at her back, and soon she was able to get her breath again. When the doctor arrived at midnight, he told Wright that his quick remedies had saved the woman's life.

/Telephones were not common, especially in country areas, and the lack of a way to signal for help spelled disaster for families like the four people in Saskatchewan who died alone, without help. Another nearby family got around the communication problem by attaching a white flag to a long pole and nailing the pole to a corner of their house, but when help did come, two members of that family had already died./

Claresholm, Alberta, which had been without a hospital since 1912, requisitioned the three-storey main building of the School of Agriculture for temporary premises. Richard Henker, who had a seven-passenger Studebaker with jump seats, drove people to the "hospital" with the sickest lying flat on the pullmanized front seat and the others, wrapped in blankets, sitting up in the back. His chief concern was to keep the patients warmly wrapped up and to get them safely up the awkward climb to the second or third floor, praying all the time that the ride to hospital — sometimes a long one — had not been too arduous.

People helped in whatever way they could. In Regina, nurses needing transportation from one part of the city to another were invited to call 5101, a special fire department number, for a ride in the chief's car or other fire department cars not required for duty. And in Kitchener-Waterloo, Ontario, car owners turned their vehicles over to the Imperial Order Daughters of the Empire, the Victorian Order of Nurses, and other organizations that rendered assistance to the sick.

The efforts of volunteers did not go unappreciated or unthanked. In Toronto, the Neighborhood Workers' Association received a touching letter of thanks for broth sent to the family of a man whose wife was trying to care for him and run the family's small cigar store as well. It concluded with these words: "I will keep an account of what you sent me and will pay you honestly. A returned man is grateful for a service rendered him like this morning. I am grateful from the bottom of my heart."

In Toronto, too, the *Globe* reported splendid work being done among Jewish families by the Orde Street Centre, "manned by Jewish women who know how to meet the Jewish food requirements. The Jewish Dispensary is in co-operation with the Senior Council of Jewish Women, and the Montefiore Patriotic Society, under the presidency of Mrs. Goldstein, is supplying pyjamas and pneumonia jackets."

Members of the Junior League in Montreal turned out to help. The Anglican chaplain at the Guards Emergency Hospital said: "You should have seen how those girls worked, and under *very* trying circumstances."

Volunteer helpers were often faced with difficult situations. Vivian Palola Kew of White Lake, British Columbia, thirteen that year, encountered one elderly couple so frightened of the germ that they wouldn't let her into the house until she had drunk a cup of very strong hot coffee, heavily laced with mustard. "They thought it would kill any germ I might have on me and I'm pretty sure it did."

Another teacher/volunteer, Esther Wilks Ozburn Dickson, cared for a sick woman on the outskirts of Vancouver. When her patient began to feel better and expressed a desire for strengthening chicken broth, eighteen-year-old Esther had to go right to the source for the ingredients. "In those days many people kept a few chickens, rabbits or bantam hens in the yard. So I toured the neighborhood until I found a place where chickens were penned; an old man (to me), who appeared quite weak, came out and said I could have a chicken if I could catch and kill it." The slaughter was no small undertaking for her but she managed it, and cleaned the chicken and made the broth.

Her next job was to care for three childen whose mother was in hospital and father, overseas. The house was so dirty that she ate her lunch outside where, although it was a relief to get out of the house, she couldn't avoid seeing the never-ending stream of funeral processions passing toward Mountain View Cemetery.

When the emergency was over, Esther Wilks returned to teaching in a one-roomed school on Westham Island, at the mouth of the Fraser River. To get there she went from her Vancouver home by ferry from Woods Landing to Ladner and across several bridges. "The farm where I was boarding was protected by mud dikes on which I walked to and from school. In the evenings I could look at the hundreds of lights bobbing up and down on the Fraser River. These were from the fishing boats, mostly Japanese, which anchored there ready for early morning. From my bedroom window I could see these boats coming to the mother boat and, with a long pike pole, land the fish to be taken to the cannery."

A young Edmonton woman, educated at Alberta and Ontario private schools, took course after course throughout the years of the war in the hope she could do something to help. No-one seemed to need her assistance with the war effort, aside from rolling bandages and knitting socks, and she wanted to do more. When the 'flu came to Edmonton, Dr. Heber C. Jamieson, acting director of bacteriology while Dr. A.C. Rankin was overseas, became immersed in the problem of epidemic control. A friend of the girl's family, he knew that she had learned to type, so he asked her to help prepare and distribute literature to the public. Her chief role at the beginning was to read what he wrote and then explain it back to him; it was assumed that if it was clear to her, it would also be clear to everyone else. Then she typed up the instructions for 'flu care and prevention, and turned them over to a staff of nine or ten men, who prepared and folded circulars to be sent to municipal secretaries around the province.

Another part of her job was to keep track of the spread of influenza across the northern areas. As reports came in, she marked the newly attacked zones with red thumbtacks, and this information was then reported to care agencies. She marvelled at the isolated neighborhoods which got the infection, places where it seemed unlikely there would have been any contact with the outside world.

Later, her involvement became more personal. "A friend and I were asked to help out in the temporary 'flu ward set up on the top floor of the Hotel Macdonald, where travellers who had been taken ill had to stay until they were well. We were giggly and excited at the prospect, but we soon discovered it was not a romantic undertaking."

The doctor, overworked to the point of exhaustion, led them through the five or six rooms where the stranded travellers lay, most of them elderly, bewhiskered men. "Just bathe them and make them comfortable," he said. "They're going to die anyway." He left the two girls, suddenly sobered by the responsibility, in charge. One man was particularly ill. When his temperature reached 104 degrees, they panicked and ran down to the lobby to telephone the doctor. "There's nothing you can do, he's probably going to die anyway," was the tired response. "You'll just have to roll his body out into the hall."

The man didn't die, however. All through the night the girls bathed him and kept his head cool, and in the morning he was better. Hardly able to believe it, they were happy and proud to report their success to the doctor when he came. The doctor praised them, and the man himself, when he was back on his feet, made a point of getting in touch with them to say thanks.

Alliance, Alberta, southeast of Edmonton, fought out the epidemic in total isolation. With the town's only doctor the first

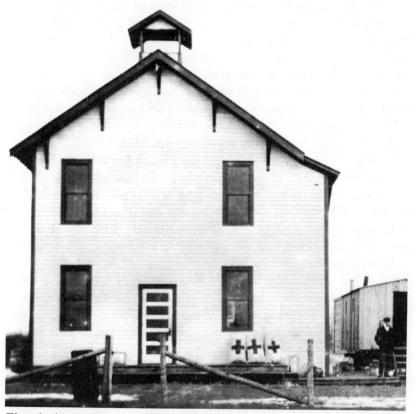

The school at Alliance, Alberta was used as a temporary hospital during the epidemic. (Photo courtesy Elizabeth Vaughan James)

fatality to the 'flu, they relied upon the St. John Ambulance training the wife of the minister had had; under her direction, and that of her husband, the school was turned into a temporary hospital.

Elizabeth Vaughan James took on the job of preparing food for the patients and staff. Working from a cook-car drawn up near the school, for nearly two months she did all the cooking except for special gifts sent by townspeople. She kept a big pot of beef broth simmering on the stove. To her mother, who worried about her and wanted her to come home, she replied, "I volunteered, and I'm old enough to decide."

To show their appreciation, the town sent a special Christmas dinner for the volunteers and those patients who could eat. Along with it was a purse of money to thank the volunteers. When patients recovered and went home, they often sent a box of chocolates to the volunteer nurses, and when Lizzie Vaughan pointed out good-naturedly that, being in the cookhouse and an unseen helper, she was missing out on the goodies, the minister sent her a letter that read: "To Whom it May Concern: This is to certify that Elizabeth Ann Vaughan has duly completed her course in cooking and is this day graduated from the Alliance Emergency Hospital. Signed and sealed this 26th day of November, 1918, by R. Clegg."

"It was a time of the Golden Rule," she says. "Everyone did something to help."

When the epidemic recurred in January 1919, Lizzie Vaughan again took up her post. Nurses came from Edmonton but they didn't stay; some took jobs in private homes, others went back to the city. And the volunteers plodded on, until the epidemic burned itself out at last in Alliance.

When a shipment of anti-'flu vaccine was sent to Dr. William Sutherland, a member of the British Columbia provincial parliament and physician to the Canadian Pacific Railway at Revelstoke, it was marked with the instruction that it be used for railway people only. The doctor read the note, looked thoughtful for a moment, then said: "I guess the other people here have a right to live as well as the CPR folks — give it to all who come."

Readying the vaccine and administering it was a difficult task. Radha Gardner Leonard, nurse-in-training, held the tiny vials of concentrated fluid in her hand and shook them for eight to ten minutes, sometimes shaking four at once to save time and energy. Because the injections had to be made deep into the large hip muscles, the needles were about the size of large darning needles and not every patient was able to take it well. Tall, husky men fainted and had to be lifted into bed.

On Christmas Eve, 1918, the nurses at Revelstoke made an attempt at normalcy in a very abnormal world by planning a scaled-down version of their usual Christmas celebration. After getting their patients well settled and comfortable, and telling them to ring if they needed anything, they went along the hall to the nurses' lounge. After only a few minutes all the bells began to ring furiously. The nurses ran at top speed back to the ward to find one of the beds empty — the patient had gone berserk, threatening to kill everyone and declaring that they were German spies. He was found outside, wandering barefoot through the snow in the hospital grounds, and he was brought back to bed. No sooner was he resettled than he became violent again, hurling flower pots at the other patients. Luckily he missed, but he did manage to break a large plate-glass window before he could be calmed with a powerful sedative. Hospital personnel called a friend of the man to sit with him, and the poor fellow, in a period of calm, begged his friend to stay to ensure that he would do no harm to the nurses who had treated him so kindly.

Children helped too. In Qu'Appelle, Saskatchewan, eight-year-old Clifford Peart struck out at 8:30 every morning with a large oval copper tub filled to the brim with hot, nourishing soup made by his mother. He loaded it on the toboggan pulled by his dog Brownie, resplendent in new harness, and with great care to avoid spills, the two made their way across the railway tracks to the school, which had been turned into a temporary hospital. There was a heavy cover of snow, and the air was cold. "The long inclined approach to the crossing was a toughie, but with Brownie pulling and me pushing, we made it. Then there was a careful look for trains and over we went to begin the descent. Now it was Brownie's duty to keep the load going straight and mine to hold it back to prevent the hot contents from running into him. We never had a mishap that I can recall." At the "hospital," strong arms relieved them of their load. When he reached home Clifford's mother would ask anxiously, "Who took the soup today?" Sadly, the turnover of helpers was high.

After another trip with the toboggan, this time to the butcher shop to pick up meat and bones for the next day's soup (along with a parcel of treats for Brownie), Peart would join the other children around the town — where there were quarantine signs on every second door — to deliver mail, empty ashpans, carry water, and split wood for people too sick to manage on their own.

One of the many truly valiant volunteers was John Hudson of Peace River, Alberta. Hugh Scott, who had moved with his family to the area from Ontario that year, was sick for two weeks and bedridden in his home as were his parents, sister, and a bachelor neighbor. He recalls: "John Hudson did not take the 'flu himself, and he was credited with saving about half of us.

"It was late January of 1919, the snow was deep and travel almost non-existent.

"John Hudson had a gruelling line of some eighteen miles that he travelled daily to keep people going. He fed everyone's horses and cows, split and carried wood to keep each family warm and melted snow to provide a meagre amount of water for everyone. He was gaunt and worn by the time people were up and about again."

Preventatives
and Cures

Every household had its own trusted preventative and remedy. Cotton bags holding a lump of camphor and worn on a cord around the neck were commonplace, and so were mothballs. Some people put their faith in violet-leaf tea, goose-grease poultices, garlic buds, castor oil, salt water snuffed up the nose, or hot coals sprinkled with sulphur or brown sugar and carried through the house accompanied by clouds of billowing smoke. A sip of oil of cinnamon allowed to seep around the tonsil area could do no harm, or one could try a mixture of warm milk, ginger, sugar, pepper, and soda for a soothing drink.

A nurse at the Kodak Company in Toronto recommended a gargle made of three drops of crude carbolic in a glass of water, and Alex Strachan, who lived on Prince Arthur Street in Montreal, always carried a handkerchief soaked in eucalyptus when he took the streetcar downtown to St. James Street. Although his family teased him, he persevered with the practice and, indeed, never caught the 'flu.

There were many theories about the most effective mixtures for chest poultices: bran, as hot as you could stand; lard, mixed with camphor and chloroform; and a half-and-half mix of lard and turpentine. When Prince Edward Island drugstores ran out of camphorated oil, one family dissolved solid camphor and mixed it with olive oil for a chest rub.

Prevent the "Flu"

by wearing

Dr. Chase's Menthol Bag

SINCE 1510 influenza has periodically swept over the known world. The last big epidemic in this country was in 1889, when almost every person in every home was brought down.

But the present form, known as Spanish "Flu" because it started in Spain, seems to be a most fatal variety on account of the quickness with which it develops into bronchial-pneumonia.

Hence the wisdom of preventing infection by every means possible, and our suggestion is to "Wear a Menthol Bag."

We have arranged for the manufacture of thousands of these Menthol Bags, and while they last shall give them away to the first persons who send in the coupon printed below.

These bags are pinned on the chest outside of the underwear, and the heat from the body causes the menthol fumes to rise and mingle with the air you breath, thereby killing the germs and protecting you against Spanish influenza and all infectious diseases.

It was always the aim of Dr. Chase to serve his fellowman by the prevention of disease whenever possible, so that this gift is in line with the policy which he established.

In his large Receipt Book Dr. Chase devoted five pages to the treatment of influenza, and of his medicines on the market Dr. Chase's Syrup of Linseed and Turpentine and Dr. Chase's Nerve Food are used to splendid advantage in fighting this malady.

The Linseed and Turpentine should be used freely just as soon as there is any tendency for the throat and bronchial tubes to be affected.

Dr. Chase's Nerve Food is used to strengthen the action of the heart and aid in the restorative process.

The great secret of keeping healthy as well as of regaining strength after illness is by keeping the blood pure, rich and red.

Red blood is the greatest of germicides, for no disease can make any great headway so long as the blood is in condition to restore the wasted tissues.

In Dr. Chase's Nerve Food are found the vital substances which go to the formation of new, rich blood. It fortifies the system against attack and hastens recovery. You can buy half a dozen boxes from your druggist for $2.75, but be sure to see the portrait and signature of A. W. Chase, M.D., on the box you buy.

But in the meantime send for a "Menthol Bag" and do all you can to protect yourself against the Spanish "Flu."

Coupon for

Dr. Chase's Menthol Bag

This coupon is good for one Dr. Chase's Menthol Bag. Kindly enclose five cents in stamps to pay cost of mailing and postage. Address Edmanson, Bates & Co. Ltd., Toronto.

Name.................................... Address....................................
                                                                          134

Manufacturers and retailers were quick to turn the epidemic to their advantage wherever possible. (The Leader, Regina, Saskatchewan, October 19, 1918. Photo courtesy Saskatchewan Archives Board)

Some swore by the salves and cough elixirs sold door-to-door by Watkins and Rawleigh men,* and drugstores did a land-office business in patent medicines. One wholesale drug company that normally sold six thousand bottles of cough medicine a week now faced a demand for three thousand bottles a day. One ounce of camphor gum sold through Eaton's catalogue in the fall and winter of 1917-18 cost ten cents, and by the time the fall/winter 1918-19 catalogue came out, the price was up to fifteen cents. Epsom salts cost ten cents a pound, castor oil was two ounces for ten cents, and the wild leaf called boneset (*Eupatorium perfoliatum*) was two ounces for a nickel. Many advertisers seized the opportunity before them. Lengthy discourses, reading for all the world like medical advisories, turned out to be ads for patent medicines. Bicycle manufacturers capitalized on the advice of doctors to get out in the fresh air.

A man working in the New Brunswick woods became ill suddenly and had to walk home three-and-a-half miles on the ice. When William Harding finally completed the journey, his aunt made a plaster for his chest, using fir-tree spills, mutton tallow, and mustard; the fir-tree spills had a healing effect and helped to take the pain away.

An Alberta recipe for a poultice ran thus: "Peel ten pounds of onions (for an adult), run them through a meat-chopper with the finest cutter available, put the ground onions into a large dish-pan; add about six or seven pounds of fine salt, stir together on the stove until it is too hot to hold in the hand. Add enough flour to thicken, just so the juice will not run." The recipe went on to describe the double vest used to hold this mixture, covered on the outside with oilcloth to avoid seepage onto the bedclothes, and it concluded with this advice: "The poultice should be kept on . . . not to exceed ten hours; then remove the poultice and rub with soft, dry towels, then with sweet oil and alcohol."

Although acetylsalicylic acid had been extracted for thousands of years from the bark of the willow tree, its modern form was not yet the household word it is today; people were just beginning to

---

*Agents for the J.R. Watkins Medical Co. and Rawleigh Products Inc. They sold spices, extracts, and remedies door-to-door in Canada from 1915 on.

use aspirin (*a* for the acetyl group and *spir* for the plants of the spirea family, containing salicylic acid). Patented by the Bayer Company, it was available in powder form from 1900 until 1917, when tablets were sold for the first time.

At Kamloops, British Columbia, an English-born second-hand dealer wandered through the town collecting old rags, bottles, and clothing. Whenever he heard that someone in a house had 'flu, he would advise: "Give 'im jalap [a powerful purgative herb] — get a road through 'im." It became a family joke for one family, the

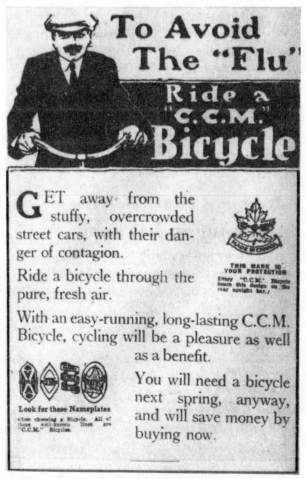

To Avoid The "Flu"

Ride a "C.C.M." Bicycle

GET away from the stuffy, overcrowded street cars, with their danger of contagion.

Ride a bicycle through the pure, fresh air.

With an easy-running, long-lasting C.C.M. Bicycle, cycling will be a pleasure as well as a benefit.

Look for these Nameplates when choosing a Bicycle. All of those well-known lines are "C.C.M." Bicycles.

You will need a bicycle next spring, anyway, and will save money by buying now.

Toronto bicycle dealers made the most of doctors' advice to get out into the fresh air. (The Globe, Toronto, October 18, 1918. Photo courtesy Ontario Archives)

Haughtons, and for years after, whenever someone felt a little off-color, the suggestion was bound to come: "Give 'im jalap, get a road through 'im!"

The Cowan family of Biggar, Saskatchewan kept a can of Creoline and water boiling on the stove day and night, and George H. Biddle, a Vancouver glazier and window washer who was constantly in contact with the public, and whose family was all down with 'flu, believed he kept himself safe by sprinkling a bit of powdered sulphur into his shoes every morning before leaving the house.

A Boston man suggested a novel approach. Perhaps, he thought, the problem was clothing put "on an animal by nature naked. The skin is a true breathing organ; its millions of blood vessels are forever gasping for air under the lightest of drapery. . . ."

There were no doctors at the Little Pine Reserve in Saskatchewan, but there were Indian remedies handed down for generations. Some who never caught the disease credited a root called wild ginger or muskrat food growing in the muskegs of the north. The Reverend Adam Cuthand, who lived through the epidemic, says: "To soothe sore throats you can grind it up and make a drink, or keep it in the side of your mouth and once in a while take a bite; the juice will trickle down your throat."

Indians of Alberta's Peace River country depended on the inner bark from the cottonwood and poplar trees, wild ginseng, yarrow and other roots, and wild cranberry bark. At Maniwaki, Quebec, Marguerite Brascoupe Budge took a mixture of skunk musk and alcohol, in proportions of one drop to half an ounce; it was mixed by her mother, who put it in vials for family and friends as a preventative. Residents of the Cumberland House Reserve in Saskatchewan relied on a mixture made this way: "Dip the end of a needle into the scent gland of a skunk, stir it into a glass of water, and drink."

A remedy based on skunk oil got a nine-year-old girl in The Pas, Manitoba into trouble with her mother and sisters. A trapper who had killed a skunk and rendered its fat into oil gave a quart sealer of the oil to Joe Poirier, who was coming down with 'flu, and told him to rub it on externally. At home his sister Florence heard someone say it was good medicine, but missed the word "external." "I took a taste and I liked it — rather like pork drippings," she remembers. Her doctoring was stopped in a hurry when she administered the cure to her sisters and their indignant reports reached their mother's ears.

Verna Robinson Prosser remembers hearing that a salt herring tied around the neck would cure a sore throat. Her grandmother, in New Brunswick, had another favorite remedy for that malady. She gathered and dried the leaves of hop vines, then steeped them in vinegar. Pressed damp against the skin, they had a soothing effect.

Mistakes were made, perhaps only amusing in retrospect. A New Brunswick doctor's wife, frantically busy helping her husband with his practice, told the maid to take a glass of cider to soothe her step-daughter's sore throat. Then, just as Dorothy Morehouse Branscombe had gulped it down gratefully, Mrs. Morehouse came running to say the maid had brought vinegar in error.

Donald Taylor was a sophomore at Mount Allison University in Sackville, New Brunswick, when fellow students began coming down with 'flu. One of them, having heard that hydrogen peroxide was an effective germ-killer, thought he would take extra precautions, so he bought a bottle of the liquid and drank as much of it as he could. Frothing and bubbling, he was rushed to the infirmary and luckily survived the drastic self-medication. Fortunately, too, he recovered from the influenza he caught a week later despite the peroxide.

In many communities, including Calgary, Alberta, citizens were required to wear gauze masks whenever they were out of their own homes. On a downtown street corner seventeen-year-old George Cardiff was reprimanded by a burly policeman for allowing his mask to slip down around his neck. "Get that mask on!" commanded Jack McGuinness. The police had their orders to enforce the law, and they did. Miscreants were fined one dollar and costs in spite of a variety of ingenious excuses. One man explained that he had been fixing a stove in front of his second-hand store and had taken off his mask so it wouldn't get dirty; another, who had just recovered from 'flu, said his doctor had advised him that wearing a mask could be injurious to his health. Neither story impressed the magistrate.

Also in Calgary, between 475 and 500 Chinese people from the city and from as far away as Regina were treated by Hong Chin of

Seattle, Washington. It was claimed that although some of the people who came from a distance were almost dead when they got there, he lost no patients. Hong Chin's method consisted of two parts: first, he located the germ, punctured the skin at that point, and applied a vegetable powder which would kill the germ; second, he removed the dead germs from the body. The report in the *Oxbow* (Saskatchewan) *Herald* did not explain how he achieved the second step, but it did report that a white man who watched the treatment requested that Hong Chin be allowed to practice for

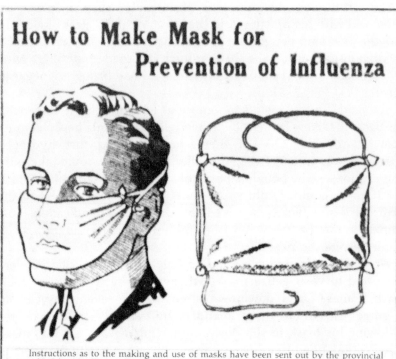

How to Make Mask for
Prevention of Influenza

Instructions as to the making and use of masks have been sent out by the provincial board of health. These are to be used when taking care of influenza patients and beginning on Thursday morning on all trains and street cars in the province. Here is the method of making the mask, published in The Bulletin some days ago and here repeated by request.

To Make a Mask — Take a piece of ordinary cheesecloth, 8 x 16 inches. Next fold this to make it 8 x 4 inches. Tie cord about 10 inches long at each corner. Apply over mouth and nose as shown in the picture.

To be worn in the sick room when taking care of the patient and on street cars and railway trains.

Keep the nose and mouth covered while coughing or sneezing.

A mask should not be worn more than two hours.

Home-made gauze masks were easy according to this explanation in the Edmonton Bulletin. *(Photo courtesy E. Brown Collection, Provincial Archives of Alberta)*

money should his claims be proved. The request was referred to the minister of health.

The Chinese cook and orderly at the hospital in High River, Alberta, believing that bloodletting would be a good preventative, scratched their wrists with pennies until the blood flowed. Neither got the 'flu/

At Qu'Appelle, Saskatchewan, the postmaster put his faith in the wreaths of pipe smoke he kept swirling around his head. Another believer in the benefits of tobacco was Toronto auctioneer Walter Ward-Price, who was constantly in and out of houses where people were sick and, on at least one occasion, entered a house where someone lay dead. A chain-smoker, he was asked by a streetcar conductor to take the cigarette out of his mouth. "Show me proof that it won't keep me safe from the 'flu," he said, then added with a grin, the cigarette still in his mouth, "I've got shoes on my feet but I'm not walking, am I?"

Dr. John Hunter, in his article "The Recent Influenza Epidemic," published in the *Canadian Practitioner and Review* of December 1918, indicated that he would not have agreed with people who favored the use of tobacco. "The amount of work done by physicians who are in the latter half of the sixth, in the seventh, and even in their eighth decade was most amazing. Old age seemed no handicap at all. It was the younger men who first showed symptoms of fatigue. Is it their morbid addiction to the cigarette that made them show up so badly in a contest with veterans?"

Some British doctors, for the first time ever, permitted smoking in war plants, and Australian pathologists smoked their pipes while conducting autopsies. A Dutch grocer went so far as to require that his employees smoke cigars on the job; the one man who refused the order was the only one to remain well. *Popular Science* magazine showed readers how to smoke even when they were required to wear a mask, by cutting a hole in the gauze and plugging it with a cork when not smoking.

Some families fumigated their houses by setting sulphur alight. According to Dr. William Oliver of Saskatoon, it was a harmful practice. "The fumes irritate the mucous membrane of the nose and throat and give an opportunity for bacteria to get in. When the nose and throat have been pained in any way, they are more susceptible to infection."

At Stearn's Son & Co. general store, at the juncture of Main and Chapel streets in Souris, Prince Edward Island, employees were instructed to be extra cautious about hygiene. They washed their hands frequently with a disinfectant soap and kept pieces of camphor ice in all the money tills. On Saturdays eight-year-old Roy White, whose father was head clerk, went to the store to help out; he remembers containers of water well strengthened with sulpha naphtha on top of all the stoves and on the furnace grates on the floor. At home, the Whites ate a candy-like mixture of onions and molasses baked on large flat pans and wore little blocks of camphor ice on cords around their necks.

The wearing of camphor bags was not a new idea according to William Perkins Bull in his book *From Medicine Man to Medical Man*. It had been used to ward off the germs of cholera in the mid-1800s, and fifty years before that, in England, it was believed that camphor would stifle the passions and quiet the nerves.

John May sold bread door-to-door in Toronto, from a horse-drawn wagon displaying a colorful picture of a woman holding a loaf over her head. The caption underneath advertised, "This is the loaf that stopped Mother baking," and children had written under that with chalk, "Yes, it killed her." May noticed that the people who bought a lot of bread, which sold for five cents a loaf, didn't seem to catch the 'flu. "I told them it was the good bread they were eating and maybe it was, but now I think about it I'm beginning to believe that people who eat simply do best."

One morning, when May made his first call of the day on Ossington Avenue, he was given a preventative the contents of which are still a mystery to him. "This fellow was a Canadian Indian who made herbal medicines. He used to make a remedy he called Mother's Friend, the best thing you ever saw for children when they got a cough. That particular day he asked me to wait a minute, and came back carrying a glass with about an inch of liquid in it. 'Drink this or you're going to be sick,' he said. Of course I didn't want to offend him so I drank it, and you know, I never got the 'flu. I'll never forget it."

A woman in Oklahoma believed that having your teeth removed would keep you safe, another in Kitchener, Ontario thought an appendectomy was a sure preventative, and young people in Philadelphia were advised to kiss only through a handkerchief. Chicago's health commissioner recommended: "Salute! Don't shake hands! When you shake hands with a friend you are actually handing him a handful of influenza and pneumonia germs." In Washington, D.C., Major Victor Vaughan estimated that if each person was in close contact with only ten others every day, and each of those with another ten, the contacts could multiply like a chain letter to a million people a week. Captain George T. Palmer, with the U.S. Sanitary Corps, decided to test the theory a little more closely. He counted the number of times in a normal day a person might touch something such as the back of a chair, money, a pen, or a door; the total came to 119 possible contacts.

Telephone company employees who had to install telephones in infected households wore cheesecloth masks soaked in formaldehyde. Sometimes, if the danger seemed very great, they would fasten the telephone to a board and push it in through a window.

There was a new public awareness of hygiene. Toronto's Union Station, which had always provided a tin drinking cup at the water tap, converted to the use of paper cups; Toronto military hospitals began sterilizing the mouthpieces of all telephones; and the chairman of the Court of Revision in Toronto told people taking the oath that they need no longer kiss the Bible, only hold it in their hands. Edmonton abolished the use of sidewalk spittoons. Fines were instituted for coughing and sneezing without covering the mouth.

A leading lung specialist advocated that people eat three cakes of yeast a day as a preventative, but his suggestion was scorned by other doctors. People baked incoming letters in the oven to kill germs; a family at Houlton, Maine did the same thing with a catalogue borrowed from a general store, and took it out nicely crisped around the edges. Recipients of a parcel of clothing from an infected household in Quebec all developed 'flu.

A legacy of the epidemic was faith in certain cures, or perhaps they just became habit. Descendants of a Montreal family who began buying bottled water in 1918, just in case tap water might carry the infection as some believed, grew to like the taste and still buy bottled drinking water more than sixty years later.

Anne Merrill, one of Canada's early women war correspondents, placed her faith in a cure she heard about by chance.

From her base in London, England she filed stories to a number of Canadian dailies on both the war and on the ravages of the epidemic. "Walking down the Strand, I saw two or three persons drop and they were rushed by ambulance to the hospital." Later, during a tour of the storerooms under the Port of London docks, she was taken to a large storage area called the Cinnamon Room. Her guide told her that the three hundred people who worked in that area had not contracted the 'flu, while there had been victims in all other parts of the storage facilities. It was enough to convince her and, until her death at the age of one hundred years, she made sure to have a pinch of cinnamon in her food every day. "Cinnamon is so simple and cheap. . . . I take a dash daily and have not had a cold in years," she said.

Another Canadian who found himself clinging to an early habit is the Reverend G.C. Salamon, OMI, who cared for the sick at his seminary in Edmonton during the fall of 1918 and suffered the disease himself during the third wave the following January. After being ordained, his first assignment was at the Holy Ghost Parish in Winnipeg, where he was told that the people in the north end of the city, mostly of central European extraction, had had a certain immunity to the disease. Perhaps, it was conjectured, it was because they included in their diet a generous proportion of onion and garlic. Although he doesn't know of a medical basis for the claim, at eighty-five years he still makes it a point to include both onion and garlic in his own diet — just to be on the safe side.

Leroy Poole, a member of the black community at Chatham, Ontario, was seventeen the year of the 'flu. "The winter of 1918-19 was very severe; people thought the wet fall had something to do with the epidemic." He didn't catch 'flu and says: "My mother used goose grease and turpentine mixed like a salve, sometimes she made a poultice out of it. I think it really helped. She told me it did, so I had to believe it!"

There was always camphor in the Poole house when Leroy was a child, and herbs gathered from the bush. "There used to be a wild leaf about four feet high which the old folks called boneset; it had a leaf something like sage but larger; and it smelled something like sage too. You could make a tea out of that to make you sweat. It was bitter and I used to run from it, but Mother would run me down and make me drink it."

Arguments raged between the open-air and closed-window factions of the population. Vancouver's medical officer of health advised people to keep their windows open, and Dr. Wesley Wallwin of Barons, Alberta, believed so strongly in the virtues of open air that he set up beds for his patients on top of hayracks. The Massachusetts State Department of Health went so far as to produce and distribute plans for a twenty-bed "shack construction open-air hospital," to ensure that patients had direct sunshine and constant outdoor air.

Voices were raised on the other side too, demanding to know how, if the germ was not borne on the wind, people in remote areas caught it? A ditty popular at the time shared their view:

> There was a little bird
> Its name was Enza
> I opened the window
> And in-flu-enza.

To quarantine or not to quarantine was another dilemma. It was up to each municipality to decide whether or not to placard infected households and while many did so, just as many thought it was not practical. Western towns, having watched the experiences of their eastern neighbors, sometimes went even farther and closed ranks entirely against outsiders by quarantining the whole town.

The topic that caused the most disagreement, however, was the use of alcohol as a cure. One commentator said that if you had had 'flu and had taken alcohol and had recovered, of course you would be in favor of it, and the people who had never used it were not equipped to make a judgment. Those who, for various reasons, opposed its use, were vehement and vocal. The wartime conservation order-in-council forbidding the use of precious foodstuffs for the distillation of liquors except for medicinal, religious, and scientific purposes meant that doctors who wished their patients to have alcohol had to write prescriptions for it. Vancouver doctors charged two dollars for these prescriptions, and a Lethbridge, Alberta man noted that doctors who prescribed whisky got more calls than those who advocated castor oil. Ottawa's Mayor Harold Fisher ventured the guess that fully half of these requests were not for truly medicinal purposes, adding darkly: "When attacked by sickness, the men addicted to excessive use of liquor are the first to go under." One doctor, who had little faith in alcohol, suggested that instead of drinking it, patients should bathe in it when suffering from 'flu. Supporters said it not only calmed the nerves, but soothed the overpowering ache in every part of the body that accompanied the malaise.

Mary Macdonald Campbell, secretary to the chief inspector of the Standard Bank, worked on the sixth floor of Calgary's Grain Exchange Building. She was startled one day when a disreputable looking man wandered in from the hall demanding a "per" (a prescription for liquor). Another secretary, who was less than five feet tall and under one hundred pounds, ordered him out. "You look to me like a bad egg," he told her, and turning to the others in the room, added, "And you don't look no better." He was finally eased out the door and directed to a nearby doctor's office; perhaps he got his "per" there.

People in Kingston, Ontario, finding little to laugh about, got some wry amusement from news of the big ward for elderly chronic alcoholics at the Hotel Dieu Hospital. "There wasn't one case of 'flu amongst them," one Kingstonian remembers. "We decided they were so preserved in alcohol that they couldn't catch anything."

Vancouver's Dr. Henry Milburn, who prescribed generous doses of brandy for a local fire chief, got a chilly reception from the man's wife when he called next morning. Not only had the fire chief stayed awake singing all night and had got no sleep, no-one else in the house had been able to sleep either.

Dr. O.E. Morehouse, the only doctor in an eighteen-mile area near Fredericton, New Brunswick, telephoned to the city for orders of whisky to be sent via the brakeman on the train. Once, when the precious consignment was delivered to the little siding, he said: "Thank God it's here at last. If only I had had a teaspoonful earlier, I could have saved a child."

Dr. Morehouse's belief was shared by many, including Dr. Matthew Robert Blake, who, speaking as a medical doctor and Conservative member of parliament representing Winnipeg North, commented in a House of Commons debate on May 21, 1919, "Although I am a temperance man, I would not want to practise medicine during such an epidemic as we had last winter without using whisky profusely upon any of my patients who were suffering from influenza. I am satisfied that the results of my treatment will compare with those of any other practitioner on this continent, and I used heaps of toxine and whisky. . .

On Prince Edward Island, prohibition commissioners voted to allow physicians living five miles or more from a vendor to act as temporary vendors, and to allow clergymen to write prescriptions for liquor.

Irma Hunter Taylor, who lived at Bassano, Alberta, was two years old. She was kept alive through a serious attack of influenza by continuous drops of brandy given her by her father. Her high fever caused her tightly-curling black hair to fall out, and when it grew again it was straight and entirely white. As she grew older her hair gradually regained color and by the time she was twelve, it was a light honey shade. The little girl, who had walked from the age of nine months, had to learn to walk all over again when she recovered from 'flu. People living in the Gaspé Peninsula of Quebec who suffered a loss of hair after high fevers found that bear fat rubbed on their heads brought back the hair thicker than before.

Another small patient given the brandy cure was W.A. Mills of Little Current, Ontario, who was only a few months old. His father kept him near the stove for two weeks and kept feeding him little drops of brandy. Thomas Brideau of the Tabusintac area of New Brunswick, one of the many who suffered relapses after they got up, was told to take two spoonsful of gin three times a day and to hold gin in his mouth whenever he left the house.

A Midland, Ontario apprenticing pharmacist, T.E.E. Greenfield, had to send doctors' orders for prescription liquor to Toronto and await their return by registered mail on the next day's train. He remained healthy while his eight colleagues sickened, one after the other, but eventually he caught the disease himself. The doctor's instruction, "Give him half that brown bottle," was hard for Greenfield's teetotalling mother to accept. After a moment's hesitation she agreed. It was the first drink of liquor he had ever had.

John B. Withrow, who grew up in what was then country but is now midtown Toronto, had just started school on Erskine Avenue. No-one in his family caught the 'flu, perhaps because of his mother's reliance on a medication called Langdale's Essence of

Cinnamon. "A few drops turned a glass of water milky. It was probably 90 percent alcohol; I know it made the head reel."

Hundreds of Ottawans crowded into the liquor dispensary on Sparks Street, despite the two dollars doctors charged for alcohol prescriptions; on Saturday, October 19 in Toronto, patrons of the government liquor stores on Church and Dundas streets were lined up four deep. At the government dispensary on Vancouver's Cambie Street, a man whose office was directly above the store observed that there were never fewer than seventy-five people in line and frequently there were more. The wait was usually up to an hour, but it was worthwhile; for $3.25, purchasers got an imperial quart of Scotch whisky. The watcher noticed an interesting mix of classes as working women and society women in the queue became friendly over the absorbing topic of symptoms. He also noted the warm concern that developed when an elderly woman who had waited for an hour couldn't find her prescription. It was a relief to everyone in line when the slip of paper finally turned up in her pocket.

In late October, the Saskatchewan government temporarily withdrew the provisions of Section 20 of the Saskatchewan Temperance Act in order to allow druggists to sell alcohol as a medicine without a doctor's prescription. They were permitted to sell not more than eight ounces of brandy, rum, gin, or whisky, as long as they were satisfied it was for medicinal purposes; if the customer lived more than five miles from the drugstore, they were allowed to double the quantity. A Regina druggist said on October 29 that there was scarcely a drop of liquor left in any city drugstore. He expressed skepticism about the value of liquor as a cure once you had developed 'flu, but recommended it as a splendid means of breaking up a cold if taken at the very beginning.

The War Ends but the 'Flu Goes On

In the autumn of 1918, the armistice was signed at the eleventh hour of the eleventh day of the eleventh month. All but one of the telegraphers working for the Canadian Press news service were on coffee break when the big news came through so, fittingly, Ottawa was the first city in the country to announce that the war was over. As prearranged, whistles blew at industrial plants, and fire department sirens blew and church bells rang. Because of the time difference between North America and Europe, it was still early morning, but Ottawans turned out in force. Coincidentally, the ban on public meetings was scheduled to be lifted that day; however, no official ruling could have stopped the delirious crowd of several thousand citizens who gathered within the hour on Parliament Hill to sing and shout. A bonfire at the corner of Sparks and O'Connor streets stopped traffic and scorched telephone and trolley wires. The Ottawa *Citizen* for that day carried a banner headline three inches high, reading, simply: "PEACE."

It was over, but of the 626,636 Canadian military personnel who served in World War I, 59,769 had lost their lives.

Rumors of the armistice had circulated a week earlier in Winnipeg, and also in Hamilton, where overeager newspaper editors had jumped the gun and had announced the news several days too soon. These false alarms did nothing to diminish the euphoria when the great day finally did arrive. For this one day, people forgot their fears and their precautions. In areas where the ban on public assembly was still in effect and officials could only order a half holiday, impromptu parades formed with blowing whistles and blaring automobile horns. Nothing was noisy enough to express the conflicting emotions triggered by the ending of this war which was supposed to have been over by Christmas 1914. A Hamilton, Ontario milkman carried on with his deliveries, but he tied two metal ashcans to the back of his wagon to make sure that nobody along his route missed the news.

For some, the war had become such a way of life that it was hard to credit that it could actually be over. Norah Hodgson MacDowell was sitting at her desk in the office of the Patriotic Fund in Montreal, where she supervised stenographers sending out cheques to dependents of servicemen. A telephone rang and she answered it; it was her mother: "They've just phoned me from the *Gazette* to say that the war is over, the war is over!" Busy and preoccupied, she didn't take in the words. "Yes, Mother, that's nice," she answered absently. "Listen to me," her mother repeated, "THE WAR IS OVER!" She took the phone away from her ear to answer someone's question, then put it back again. "Mother, I'll be home for lunch," she said. As she hung up the

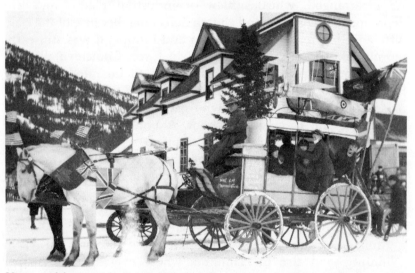

Victory celebrations at Banff, Alberta. Some merry makers are wearing gauze masks. (Photo courtesy Glenbow Archives)

phone, the impact of her mother's words struck her. She ran downstairs to the door of the building as two soldiers ran by. They shouted, "Have you heard, Miss, the war is over, the war is over!"

Elmer J. Farrish, from Huron County, Ontario, had answered the call for harvesters to help with the 1918 bumper crop in the west. His trip to Saskatchewan began when his father drove him by horse and buggy to the town of Lucknow, where he took a train to Toronto. From there west he travelled on a train made up of twenty-two colonist cars in which seats facing each other pulled out to make bunks for sleeping. He spent the autumn stooking sheaves and helping out on threshing gangs, and returned to Ontario in November on a train that made few stops because the conductor feared picking up infection. He arrived at Toronto's Union Station on Armistice Day. "Everybody was celebrating. The whistles were blowing, the bands were playing, everybody was on the streets and the shops were closed."

There were no electric signs in the station then to show train arrivals and departures, so they were announced by loudspeaker.

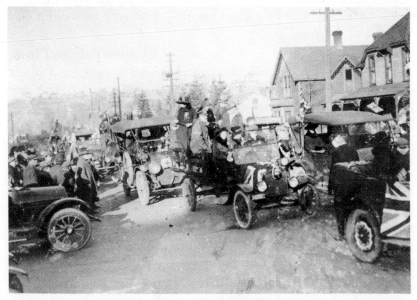

Victory parade in Calgary, Alberta. Note the policemen and others wearing gauze masks. The hill in the background is thought to be North Hill. (Photo courtesy Glenbow Archives)

"When it was almost time for the station master to make an announcement, he couldn't be heard over the racket. He approached a couple of English ladies who were banging on tin pans with sticks and told them they would have to be quiet or go outside. They really gave him a piece of their minds, called him pro-German and a lot of other things, and said if they were over 'ome they'd be able to make all the noise they liked."

Over 'ome in London, England that day, bonfires burned in Trafalgar Square. With crowds gathered outside Buckingham Palace, King George V and Queen Mary appeared on the balcony. The King said: "With you I rejoice. Thank God for the victories the allied armies have won, which have brought hostilities to an end. Peace is in sight."

In many parts of Canada, the hated Kaiser Wilhelm appeared in effigy and was well and truly destroyed. Effie Zwicker Matchett was a grade nine student at Mahone Bay, Nova Scotia, where 'flu-infected homes were placarded with large signs lettered in black with the words "Spanish Influenza," and where the schools were still closed. Early that morning, Effie and her sister heard the school bells ring. "We flew out of bed and got dressed quickly, thinking school must be going to start — then we found out it was the end of the war."

A stage was erected in the middle of Mahone Bay, and from there the ministers of all the churches, the mayor, and other dignitaries spoke to the townspeople crowded around. The day was cold and the ground frozen, but there was no snow.

The Anglican minister, the Reverend E.A. Harris, made an artistic effigy of Kaiser Wilhelm with stuffed potato sacks. This likeness was tied to the back of a wagon and hauled through town to the top of a large hill called Spion Kop. Members of the Women's Institute brought brooms and sticks and paddles, and everyone followed along behind. "They pounded the devil out of the Kaiser," Effie Matchett remembers. At Spion Kop someone started a huge bonfire, and the young people piled it high with wooden boxes; when the fire was going well, in went the effigy.

The nine children of the Lafferty family at Chipman, New Brunswick, and their mother, were all sick with influenza; churches and schools were closed. But when the CPR machine shop whistles blew on Sunday, November 10, signalling the end of the war — just a little ahead of time — the world looked suddenly brighter.

Saskatchewan farmers lit up the skies with burning straw-stacks, and everywhere hoarded liquor supplies suddenly appeared to help with the celebrations. But two Cadillac, Saskatchewan men, doing their bit to help with the merrymaking by bringing twenty-eight gallons of Montana Red Eye and three gallons of Three Star brandy across the border from the United States, were apprehended and each fined two hundred dollars and costs. "Great was the sorrow in the district when it was learned that the liquor had been seized," reported the *Morning Leader*. "Police say the shipment was awaited by a large number of thirsty citizens who were deeply chagrined when deprived of lubricant. . . ."

Regina people thronged Wascana Park for speeches and singsongs, and in Kindersley there was a parade. As William John Wolsey stood watching, he noticed the eyes of some of the people in the crowd. "They were sick, and feverish-looking." Perhaps, even knowing they should not have been out, they had to see for themselves to believe that this long, long war was really and truly finished.

The *Edmonton Journal* of October 31 headlined: "Turkey has Surrendered Unconditionally," and directly below appeared news that Alberta had not yet approached the peak of the influenza outbreak. "Epidemic Spreading Rapidly, says Minister Public Health."

Rumors of peace struck Vancouver on November 7. A week before, the city had turned out to welcome returning servicemen and, though there was still a ban on indoor meetings, the Victory Loan drive went forward with a rally, a torchlight parade, and the added attraction of Harry Gardiner, "the human fly," climbing up the outside of the Hotel Vancouver. November 11 excitement suffered not a whit from these too-early celebrations.

The day was cold and the wind brisk at Ripley, Ontario. Adelene Mooney Martyn, sixteen, was just recovering from 'flu, but so she would not miss the historic occasion, her father rented one of the two cars in the village. With the livery man driving and Adelene well bundled up against the cold, they drove downtown to see the Kaiser being burned. Fearful of germs, their friends would not come near the car but waved from a distance.

For Cecilia Cullen De Lory of Charlottetown, Prince Edward Island, November 11 has always evoked sad memories. "My mother, my older sister and four brothers were ill with 'flu. After eight days my mother, only 40 years old, got pneumonia and died. ·My father and I attended her funeral at four o'clock on November 11, 1918, to the sound of bells ringing for the Armistice."

And in Alberta, Gertrude Murphy Charters, the young VAD who nursed the miners at Drumheller, had been called out into the country. As she drove along a quiet road on the morning of November 11, she heard the bells ring to announce that peace had come, and thought: "God's in his heaven." But even then, she was on her way to take over the care of still another family sick with Spanish Influenza. The war was over, but the epidemic was not.

And in Its Wake

The epidemic was not a tidy occurrence that began on a specific date and ended on another specific date; in some parts of the country it recurred again and again. Many of the thirty thousand to fifty thousand Canadians who died of the disease were young adults who left small children. Some of those children went into orphanages, while the lucky ones became part of other families. At Kindersley, Saskatchewan, the Wolseys took a small boy into their home; he remained with the family for a year, mostly in the care of fifteen-year-old Mona Wolsey Ogle. "His mother, who was a close friend of my mother, had died in the epidemic and his father couldn't look after the little fellow and work too. When finally the father arranged to take him to his grandmother in Ontario, we were so sad," she says. They lost touch with him, but still cherish a snapshot taken just before he left.

More than thirty years after the epidemic, J.A. Kinnear, town foreman at Coleman, Alberta was asked to survey the graveyard and register all the burials. Under long grass he and his crew discovered at least twenty graves, only about four feet by two, in an oval shape, outlined by native boulders. They were the graves of children who had died in 1918.

Canadians who survived the 'flu were often left with heart trouble and respiratory weakness that made it impossible for them to pick up their lives where they had left off. Robert Gain of Dunany, Quebec was one of those. He was taken to the Montreal General Hospital in December, and when his wife went to visit him on New Year's Day she contracted 'flu. She died two weeks later, leaving five children aged between eighteen months and nine years. At first the children's grandfather stayed with them, then good neighbors took over the care of the three youngest children. Gain's recovery was very slow and when at last he came home from hospital, in March, he was unable even to feed himself; not until June was he able to walk again.

Changes to lives were enormous. On Prince Edward Island, a woman now in her eighties thinks back on the task that fell to her older sister. "When Mother died I was away from home, and my sister took over the care of all the younger ones. I don't think it ever occurred to any of them that she was giving up anything, or to thank her. They only remembered that she had to discipline them."

The poignant experience of one Canadian serviceman was probably repeated a hundredfold. After becoming engaged to marry a local girl, he was sent overseas and was wounded in battle; while convalescing in a British hospital, he fell in love with a nurse there. Back home after the war, he faced the dreadful task of telling the Canadian girl he couldn't marry her. She was deeply hurt, and the man's own family turned against him. Anguished, he wrote to the nurse in Britain to say that he could not in conscience break his original promise, but instead of a response from her, a letter came from her friend telling him that she had died in the 'flu epidemic. The friend added bitterly that at least she had been spared the knowledge of his perfidy. All of his life those lines were burned into his mind and heart.

But, despite the losses and the pain, some good came out of it all. The vast majority of Canadians who lived through the epidemic did so with courage, fortitude, and kindliness. People who worked hard to help their neighbors remember with pleasure the friends they made and, with a degree of pride, the new knowledge of their ability to cope. If their nursing skills were limited, they were stout of heart. The Spanish Lady reinforced the tradition of neighborliness and sharing that was characteristic of Canada's early years.

People who had never asked for help in their lives, and never expected to do so, forgot their pride when their families' welfare was at stake. Mortgages, something people didn't talk about if they had them, were taken out to pay for drugs. Doctors and nurses offered their services without asking for payment.

People even found ways to laugh at the 'flu. Verse writers were inspired. This rhyme, in the *Canora* (Saskatchewan) *Advertiser:*

> *A Tale of the Flu*
> A flea and a fly had the 'flu
> They neither were sure what to do
> "Let us fly," said the flea
> "Let us flee," said the fly
> So they flew through a flaw in the flue,

turned up in slightly different form under the heading "The Passing Jest" in the *Globe*, Toronto, on October 4:

> A flea met a fly in a flue
> "Let us flee," said the fly
> "Let us fly," said the flea
> But the 'flu caught the two in the flue.

When the wearing of gauze masks became the law in Alberta, an anonymous poet with the Canadian Bank of Commerce expressed his feelings this way:

> Disconsolate along the streets
> Man walks, oppressed with care
> And hopeless scans the crowd he meets
> To find his ladye faire.
> For, swathed in white from ear to ear
> She braves the dreaded 'flu
> And as he greets each unknown dear
> She answers with: "At Choo!"

A Toronto editorial writer waxed philosophical. "During the suspended animation due to the invasion of Spanish influenza, the world is permitted to think. ... This strange dispensation may prove a blessing in disguise, and to enable us to accumulate a reserve of nervous energy and thought that will be needed during the coming days of transition from a state of war into a state of peace. We need these long Sabbaths, these recuperative periods, and a world that will not take a short rest is eventually forced into a long one."

While the effectiveness of hastily-organized volunteer groups was nothing short of astounding, communities were brought face-to-face with the inadequacies of their medical facilities, and budgets were increased to allow for the building of new hospitals. A course in public health nursing was established at Nova Scotia's Dalhousie University. There had for some time been pressure from groups, including the Canadian Medical Association and the United Farm Women's Association, for increased cooperation between the provinces in the matter of public health, and for the establishment of a central health bureau. In October, 1918 a report to the vice-chairman of the War Committee of the Cabinet on the establishment of a federal department of health stated: "The recent epidemic of Spanish Influenza points to the need for a Federal Health Authority. Throughout this crisis there was no organization competent to handle the problem on a national scale. The control of the disease was necessarily left to local bodies, many of them ill-formed and all of them inevitably lacking in

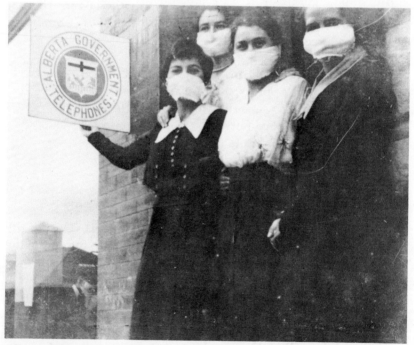

Alberta Government Telephone operators at High River defy the 'flu epidemic. (Photo courtesy Glenbow Archives)

co-ordinated effort." The bill to establish a federal department of health was given first reading in March 1919, and the department became operational that fall.

Losses to business cannot be estimated. Merchants suffered not only because people were too ill to shop, but also because shoppers hesitated to venture out into crowds. They lost, too, because of the number of staff off sick. Theatres, pool halls, restaurants, and dance halls lost heavily. Hotels in small centres found their rooms empty as travelling salesmen, the mainstay of the hotel business, either weren't taking the risk of travel or were confined to the larger centres because of the ban on travel — or because they were sick. Edmonton estimated that the direct outlay to the city for nursing equipment and supplies would add up to twenty-five thousand dollars; in addition to street railway and other losses, the total bill would be the neighborhood of one hundred thousand dollars.

Ten thousand railway workers in eastern Canada were off sick in October, and the Canadian Railway Board was forced to ask that their ex-employees in army camps be released to help get traffic moving. "Blizzards, ice, storm and zero weather last winter did not do as much damage as the Spanish Influenza is doing in impairing service in Canada," an official said.

About half the coal mines at Drumheller were shut down during October because of the heavy toll of illness and death among the miners; lignite mines at Bienfait, Saskatchewan shipped out thirty cars of coal less a day than was their norm; and a similar situation existed at Lethbridge.

Banks and farm implement companies in Manitoba reported serious difficulties on account of illness among farmers and small merchants, and remittances to wholesalers were reported to be the smallest in years.

Heavy pressure was put on telephone companies because so many customers were using telephones instead of going out, and because so many of their operators and other staff were sick. At some of the small Bell Telephone Company exchanges, four-fifths of the staff was away at one time. Former employees volunteered to help out and anyone who had ever run a switchboard pitched in.

One of the hardest-hit industries was insurance. In London, England the Prudential Assurance Company paid out more than twice as much in 'flu claims as they did in war claims. "It was just as though two large battles were going on in addition to the fighting on all fronts," their actuary said. The same was true in Canada, where in 1918 12 percent more 'flu claims were paid than war claims, and during 1919, when war claims would be expected to go down, and did, to 4.64 percent of the whole, influenza claims amounted to 17.69 percent.

On the medical front, it was clear that the vaccines produced in 1918 had not worked, and that other methods of control, such as quarantine and isolation, had been just as futile. With the crisis over, apart from isolated flareups, there was at last time for epidemiologists to study the cause of the epidemic and to track its progress. Scientists continued to search for the cause of influenza, more than ever convinced that it was a virus and not Pfeiffer's bacillus, as had once been thought.

In 1933, at the National Institute for Medical Research Farm Laboratories at Mill Hill in the suburbs of London, England, Dr. Patrick Laidlaw, and Dr. Christopher F. Andrews, who was later knighted for his work on influenza and the common cold, made a breakthrough in isolating a virus that affected not only the view of influenza but a host of other viral illnesses as well. Experimenting with ferrets, they discovered that they could take nasal secretions from humans who had influenza, drop them into the noses of the ferrets and produce the disease in the little animals. Within a month there was a full-scale epidemic among the ferrets, one of which sneezed into a researcher's face and gave him influenza. The work established that the disease had been caused by an infectious agent that could be transmitted through the air. The next step was to try the same experiment with mice; again, it worked.

Researchers in Ann Arbor, Michigan, experimented with growing the virus in fertile chicken eggs, a procedure still used today, and one that was a direct step towards developing a vaccine against the disease.

By 1940 scientists had divided the virus into two major strains, A and B, and by examining blood samples from persons who had had 'flu in 1918, they established that Influenza Virus A had been the villain in that epidemic. As well, they determined that the pneumonia which often followed the Spanish 'flu was usually produced by an association of the virus with another organism or germ, usually *Staphylococcus* or *Streptococcus*.

By that time electron microscopes were in use and the virus was finally photographed in all its glory. So tiny was each virus particle that twenty or thirty million of them would fit on the head of a pin, with room to spare.

The next question: Where did Spanish Influenza go, and could it come back again? Sir Christopher Andrewes thinks it could. "I can believe that the virus goes underground and perhaps does so all over the world, causing odd subclinical infections and not much more, but able to become active and epidemic when the time is ripe."

If that "ripe" time arrived, and we had another outbreak of the magnitude of the 1918 pandemic, how would Canada fare? In many ways, better. People in the most remote areas can communicate with others by radio telephone. There are more and larger hospitals, and social agencies to care for people without families. Federal and provincial health authorities work together. Most important, we have available diagnostic tests and preventive vaccines, and powerful antibiotics for treating bacterial complications.

Medically, then, we should have every confidence of a less terrifying and lethal situation. We can only hope that we would be as wealthy again in terms of human kindness.

Bibliography

This bibliography is an alphabetical listing of major sources. In the case of newspapers listed, a number of issues spanning the period of the 1918 influenza epidemic were used unless a specific date is given. Institutions and archives that provided material are listed at the end.

Actuarial Society of America, Chicago. Book review on *Report on the Pandemic of Influenza, 1918-19*. *Transactions* 22(1921): 541-553.

Alberta Provincial Police, Edmonton. "Annual reports for the year ending December 31, 1918."

Amherst (Nova Scotia) *News & Sentinel*, 1918.

Andrews, M. W., "Epidemic and public health: influenza in Vancouver, 1918-19." *B.C. Studies* 34(Summer 1977): 21-44.

Assiniboia (Saskatchewan) *Times*, June 15, 1955.

Barker, George. *Forty Years a Chief*. Winnipeg: Peguis Publishers Limited, 1979.

Bell Telephone Company, Montreal. "Annual report, 1918," 6-7.

Beveridge, W.I.B. *Influenza: The Last Great Plague. An Unfinished Story of Discovery*. New York: Prodist, 1977.

Bird, Michael J. *The Town that Died: A Chronicle of the Halifax Disaster.* Toronto: McGraw-Hill Ryerson Limited, 1962.

Blue Bell Magazine, Bell Canada, Montreal, 1961.

Boucher, S. "The epidemic of influenza." *Canadian Medical Association Journal (CMAJ)* 8(1918): 1087-1092.

Braithwaite, M. "The Year of the Killer Flu." *Maclean's,* February 1, 1953.

Bull, Wm. Perkins. *From Medicine Man to Medical Man: A Record of a Century and a Half of Progress in Health and Sanitation as Exemplified by Developments in Peel.* Toronto: The Perkins Bull Foundation, George J. McLeod, Ltd., 1934.

Cadham, F.T. "The use of a vaccine in the recent epidemic of influenza." *CMAJ* 9(1919): 519-527.

Calgary Canadian, 1918.

Calgary *Herald,* 1918.

Canada. Department of Indian Affairs. "Report for the year ended March 31, 1919," 42-53.

Canadian Annual Review, 1919. Toronto: Canadian Annual Review Company.

Canadian Red Cross Society, Toronto. "Annual report for year 1920."

Canora (Saskatchewan) *Advertiser,* 1918.

Cashman, Tony. *Heritage of Service: The History of Nursing in Alberta.* Edmonton: Alberta Association of Registered Nurses, 1966.

Charters, G. "The Black Death at Drumheller." *Maclean's,* March 5, 1966.

Collier, Richard. *The Plague of the Spanish Lady.* New York: Atheneum, 1974.

Colombo, John Robert. *Colombo's Book of Canada.* Edmonton: Hurtig Publishers, 1978.

Craig, John. *The Years of Agony.* Toronto: Natural Science of Canada Ltd., 1977.

Cranbrook (British Columbia) *Herald,* 1918.

Dateline Canada. Toronto: Holt Rinehart & Winston of Canada Ltd., 1967.

T. Eaton Archives, Toronto. Catalogues, 1917-19.

Edmonton Bulletin, 1918.

Edmonton Journal, 1918.

Edmonton Local Board of Health and Health Department. "History, 1871-1979," 29-32.

Encyclopedia Canadiana. Ottawa: The Canadiana Company Limited, a subsidiary of the Grolier Society of Canada Limited, 1965.

Fleming, Archibald Lang. *Archibald the Arctic.* New York: Appleton-Century-Crofts, Inc., 1956.

4th Estate, Halifax, September 22, 1976.

Gordon, Henry. "The Labrador Parson." Provincial Archives of Newfoundland and Labrador.

Gordon, Irene. "Spanish influenza in Winnipeg, 1918-19." Report for Honours History Class, University of Manitoba, February, 1981.

Grande Prairie (Alberta) *Herald,* 1918.

Graves, Charles. *Invasion by Virus: Can it Happen Again?* London: Icon Books Limited, 1969.

Halifax *Morning Chronicle*, 1918.

Hamilton (Ontario) Magazine, November, 1979.

Harbour Grace (Newfoundland) *Standard*, 1918.

Harris, T.W. Papers. Glenbow Museum, Alberta.

Heagerty, John J. *Four Centuries of Medical History in Canada*, Vol. 1. Toronto: The Macmillan Company of Canada Limited, 1928.

Heagerty, J.J. "Influenza and vaccination." *CMAJ* 9(1919): 226-28.

Hoehling, A.A. *The Great Epidemic: When the Spanish Influenza Struck.* Boston: Little, Brown and Company, 1961. Published simultaneously in Canada by Little, Brown and Company (Canada) Limited, Toronto.

Howitt, H.O. "Some observations in a recent epidemic." *The Public Health Journal* 11(1919): 508-510.

Hunter, John. "The recent influenza epidemic." *The Canadian Practitioner and Review.* 12(1918): 355-57.

Imperial Order Daughters of the Empire Archives, Toronto.

Jameson, Sheilagh S. *Chautauqua in Canada.* Calgary: Glenbow-Alberta Institute, 1979.

Kelowna (British Columbia) *Daily Courier*, November 23, 1968.

Kemp, H.S.M. *Northern Trader.* Toronto: Ryerson Press, 1956.

Kerr, Don, and Hanson, Stan. *Saskatoon: The First Half-Century.* Edmonton: NeWest, 1982.

Lancet, London, January 14, 1919.

Lapointe, Arthur. *Soldier of Quebec (1916-1919).* Translated by R.C. Fetherstonhaugh. Montreal: Editions Edouard Garand, 1931.

Leach, Brother Frederick. *60 Years with Indians and Settlers on Lake Winnipeg*. n.d., n.p.

Le Devoir, Montreal, 1918.

Le Droit, Ottawa, 1918.

MacGregor, James G. *A History of Alberta*. Edmonton: Hurtig Publishers, 1972.

Manitoba Free Press, 1918.

Marks, Geoffrey, and Beatty, William K. *Epidemics*. New York: Charles Scribner's Sons, 1976.

McCullough, John W.S. "Influenza." *The Public Health Journal* 10(1919): 28-30.

McCullough, John W.S. "The control of influenza in Ontario." *CMAJ* 8 (1918): 1084-86.

McGinnis, J.P. "A city faces an epidemic." *Alberta History* 24 (Autumn 1976): 1-11.

McGinnis, J.P. "The impact of epidemic influenza: Canada, 1918-19." The Canadian Historical Association Historical Papers (1977), 121-40.

Metropolitan Life Insurance Company, New York. *Statistical Bulletin* 57(September 1976): 3-7.

Montreal *Gazette*, 1918.

Montreal Star, 1918.

Morton, Gladys. "The pandemic influenza of 1918." *The Canadian Nurse*, Toronto, December, 1976.

Newfoundland Quarterly, St. John's, 1920.

Nicholson, G.W.L. *The White Cross in Canada: A History of St. John Ambulance*. Montreal: Harvest House, 1967.

O'Neill, Paul. *The Oldest City.* Erin, Ontario: Press Porcepic, 1975.

Ottawa *Citizen*, 1918.

Ottawa Journal, 1918.

Oxbow (Saskatchewan) *Herald*, 1918.

Payzant, Joan and Lewis. *Like a Weaver's Shuttle.* Halifax: Nimbus Publishing Limited, 1979.

Pettigrew, E. "Another day, another door." Imperial Oil *Review*, 1(1980).

Prince Rupert (British Columbia) *Daily News*, October 24, 1968.

Public Archives of Canada, Ottawa. RG 24, vols. 1847 and 4270, National Defence papers; RG 29, vol. 300, Health and Welfare records; RG 42, vol. 290, Marine records; MG 26H, vol. 94, papers of Sir Robert Borden.

Regina *Leader*, 1918.

Regina *Morning Leader*, 1918.

Royal Canadian Mounted Police, Ottawa. "Report for the year ended September 30, 1928," 57-61.

Royal Gazette Extraordinary, St. John's: J.W. Withers, King's Printer, 1918.

Saint John Globe, 1918.

St. John's *Daily News*, 1918.

Saskatoon Daily Star, 1918.

Sterling Drug Ltd., Aurora, Ontario. Leaflet: "History of Aspirin." March 18, 1981.

Swan River (Manitoba) *Star & Times,* 1918.

Swettenham, John. *Canada and the First World War.* Toronto: McGraw-Hill Ryerson, 1973.

Them Days, Labrador. 2(1975), 1(1980).

Toronto *Globe,* 1918.

Toronto Daily Star, 1918.

Toronto World, 1918.

Vancouver *Daily Province,* 1918.

Vancouver Sun, 1918, March 31, 1976.

van Rooyen, C.E., and Rhodes, A.J. *Virus Diseases of Man.* New York: Thomas Nelson & Sons, 1948.

Victoria *Daily Colonist,* 1918.

Victoria Daily Times, October 25, 1952.

Victorian Order of Nurses for Canada, Ottawa. "Chief superintendent's report, 1918."

War Cry, 1918. Salvation Army, Toronto.

Whitelaw, T.H. "The practical aspects of quarantine for influenza." *CMAJ* 9(1919): 1070-74.

Winnipeg Free Press, 1918.

Winnipeg Tribune, 1918.

Woods, Shirley E., Jr. *Ottawa, The Capital of Canada.* Toronto: Doubleday Canada Limited, 1980.

Reports, correspondence, and newspaper microfilm from:

Provincial Archives of British Columbia, Victoria;
Provincial Archives of Alberta, Edmonton;
Glenbow Museum, Calgary;
Saskatchewan Archives Board, Regina and Saskatoon;
Provincial Archives of Manitoba, Winnipeg;
Hudson's Bay Company Archives, Winnipeg;
Archives of Ontario, Toronto;
City of Toronto Archives;
Metropolitan Toronto Library;
John P. Robarts Library, and Science and Medicine Library,
    University of Toronto;
Anglican Church of Canada, Toronto;
Queen's University Archives, Kingston;
Archives Deschâtelets, Ottawa;
Canadian War Museum, Ottawa;
Canadian National Library Services, Montreal;
Osler Library, McGill University, Montreal;
Monastère de l'Hôtel-Dieu de Québec, Québec;
Archives nationales du Québec, Québec;
Provincial Archives of New Brunswick;
Public Archives of Nova Scotia;
Public Archives of Prince Edward Island;
Provincial Archives of Newfoundland and Labrador;
Memorial University of Newfoundland.
Also, reports and correspondence from provincial departments
    of health.

INDEX

New Pelican, Newfoundland, 24
Newsholme, Sir Arthur, 22
New Westminster, British
  Columbia, 75
New York, New York, 14, 19
Niagara, Ontario, 9
Nicolet County, Quebec, 46
North Portal, Saskatchewan, 61
North River, Labrador, 28

Obed, Joshua, 31
O'Brien's Limited, 53
Ogle, Mona Wolsey, 131
Okak, Labrador, 29, 31
Old Souris (*see* Ile-à-la-Crosse,
  Sask.), 81
Oliver, Dr. William, 117
Olsen, Mical, 77
Ontario board of health, 13, 51
Ontario Health Act, 54
Ottawa, Ontario, 3, 38, 53, 54, 86,
  100, 121, 124, 125
Ottawa board of health, 53
Ottawa *Citizen*, 125
Otterville, Ontario, 55
Owen, Mr., 85
Oxbow, Saskatchewan, 62
Oxbow Herald (Saskatchewan), 61,
  116

Paddon, Dr., 27
Palmer, Capt. George T., 119
Paquette, Constable, 80
Paradise Hill, Saskatchewan, 62
Paris, Ontario, 18
Parks, Dr. Arthur E., 48
Parliament of Canada, xiii, 13
Parsons, Ella, 89
Parsons, Hayward, 25
Parsons, Mrs. Hayward, 27
Patterson, Dr. Margaret, 17, 97
Peace River, Alberta, 78, 109, 114
Pearson, Dr., 14

Peart, Clifford, 108
Perrett, Rev. Walter, 29
Perry, C. C., 97
Peters, Eileen, 43
Petersen, H. E., 62
Pfeiffer's bacillus, 19
Philadelphia, Pennsylvania, 118
Pickford, Mary, 58
Pine Bluffs (*see* Cumberland
  House, Sask.), 80
Pine River, Saskatchewan, 81
Plague of Justinian, 5
Pleasantville, Nova Scotia, 102
Poirier, Florence (Gudgeon), 59,
  114
Poirier, Jean Mastai, 59
Poirier, Joe, 114
Poole, Leroy, 120
Popular Science, 117
Port Arthur, Ontario, 56
Port Dover, Ontario, 53
Port McNeill, British Columbia,
  89
Port Simpson, British Columbia,
  97
Pouce Coupe, Alberta, 102
Prince Albert, Saskatchewan, 81
Prince Edward Island, 38
Prince Edward Island education
  department, 37
Prince Rupert, British Columbia,
  75, 91, 97
Pringle, R. A., 3
Prosser, Verna Robinson, 93, 115
Prudential Assurance Company,
  135

Qu'Appelle, Saskatchewan, 108,
  117
Quebec City, Quebec, 8, 9, 10,
  42, 63
Quebec Superior Board of Health,
  20, 48